The True Diary
of a Mum-to-be

A pregnancy companion

by

Charlie Plunkett

Grosvenor House
Publishing Limited

All rights reserved
Copyright © Charlie Plunkett, 2010

Charlie Plunkett is hereby identified as author of this
work in accordance with Section 77 of the Copyright, Designs
and Patents Act 1988

The book cover picture is copyright to Charlie Plunkett

This book is published by
Grosvenor House Publishing Ltd
28-30 High Street, Guildford, Surrey, GU1 3HY.
www.grosvenorhousepublishing.co.uk

This book is sold subject to the conditions that it shall not, by way of
trade or otherwise, be lent, resold, hired out or otherwise circulated
without the author's or publisher's prior consent in any form of binding or
cover other than that in which it is published and
without a similar condition including this condition being imposed
on the subsequent purchaser.

A CIP record for this book
is available from the British Library

ISBN 978-1-907211-95-9

Also by Charlie Plunkett

The True Diary of a Bride-to-be

Coming soon...
The True Diary of Baby's First Year

Praise for Charlie Plunkett

'*Entertaining and engaging with great down to earth advice*'. **Green Baby**

'*If you're looking for a Mills & Boon view of pregnancy, then this book isn't for you, but if you're looking for a personal, honest, funny, warts-and-all diary of a pregnancy then this book is a must-buy!*' **MumsTheWord**

'*It was a joy getting to know 'Pear' and his ever increasing influence on his soon-to-be parents. This fabulous book will be a complete hit with every mum-to-be*'. **Blooming Marvellous**

'*Absolutely brilliant! This really is the essential guide for any prospective parent. It's a heart-warming, personable and factual account of what to really expect when you're expecting - emotionally as well as physically! From the first page you bond with the author and you feel like you're reading your best friend's diary*'. **Hamill Baby**

Acknowledgements

I would like to thank my wonderful husband Dave who has supported me through the highs and lows of our journey towards becoming parents. When things were tough we became even closer than ever. He has proven himself not only to be a fabulous husband but an absolute 'natural' when it comes to being a daddy. Both Cole and I are truly blessed to have him in our lives.

Thank you to all our family and friends who are a constant source of love and support to us. Especially our dear friends Nick and Catherine for helping us with the never-ending D.I.Y. on our flat before Cole arrived.

To my mum and dad, Mary and Tony, and also Dave's mum, Janet and husband Tony. I hope Dave and I will be as great as parents to our baby as you were to us. We love you all so much. Cole is a lucky baby to have such doting grandparents.

We owe so much to our wonderful HypnoBirthing teacher Karen. She took a totally neurotic and anxious mum-to-be (me!) and managed to teach me skills and techniques that helped us to have the birth we had dreamt of.

Huge thanks to our lovely doula Samsara, whose presence at Cole's birth gave us so much comfort and confidence. We will always think of her fondly for her wonderful advice in all things 'baby'.

Thanks also go to Dom; my fantastic pregnancy yoga teacher for showing me the importance of squats and pelvic floor exercises, for which I shall be eternally grateful!

Finally, I mustn't forget my marvellous editor Stefanie, for her attention to detail, patience and ability to explain to me that sometimes less is more when it comes to the use of an exclamation mark!

To Dave with lots of love from your wife, you are mine and Cole's hero!

To Cole aka Pear - Thank you for choosing us as your parents we are so happy to finally have met you, our little angel.

Contents

CONTENTS

Introduction

If you are reading this diary then the chances are you are either planning to get pregnant or already are - in which case congratulations are in order.

In my life I have only done two, what I consider truly grown up things. The first was to get married and the second, you guessed it, was to start a family.

Dave and I had a fantastic wedding - two actually, one in Vegas and the other at The Royal Pavilion in Brighton. Our honeymoon had been a whirlwind tour around America taking in Vegas, LA, San Francisco, Miami, Orlando and New York. It was in Disneyland that we started talking seriously about having children. I think some of that Disney magic not only brought out the inner child in us, but had us wishing that someday we would return with a child of our own.

Dave was already in his forties and I was fast approaching the big 4-0 so time was a ticking! We have both had a multitude of different jobs, from working as dancers to being extras on a film set where we met some 15 years ago. Neither of us were particularly career minded, we'd travelled quite a bit and felt that we had done all the things we wanted to before settling down. So the natural progression after getting married was to take the huge step into that unknown territory 'parenthood'. Hence our wedding photos had only just been placed in their albums and we were already starting to get in some baby making practice!

I realise now how unprepared, not to mention ignorant I was of all things baby. I rather naively had thought we would have unprotected sex and nine months later we would be parents, if only things were that simple! To be fair, I think my lack of knowledge stemmed from the fact that at school instead of taking sex education classes I had private violin lessons instead! Sadly, despite the money my parents spent on the classes, I never really grasped the instrument; suffice to say Vanessa Mae can sleep easy.

I obviously had a basic idea of the mechanics and knew how a baby was conceived, but I didn't have a clue about much else. There were so many words relating to pregnancy that I practically needed an interpreter for. Books and magazines talking about trimesters, ovulation, implantation and oxytocin, may as well have been written in another language for all the sense they made to me.

My lovely husband Dave, was very much of the opinion that not thinking about things too much and just letting nature and as he put it his, 'super sperm' take their course, would be the best way to start a family. I wish I could pinch some of his laid back attitude and calm self-assuredness. But I'm a bit of a control freak with Dot Cotton-like tendencies towards hypochondria, both traits not totally conducive to having a stress free pregnancy.

I may not have studied sex education at school but I had seen my fair share of pregnancy related story lines on television: Casualty, Doctors, Eastenders and, of course the good old Aussie soaps, Neighbours and Home and Away. All of them appeared to show that unless you got raving drunk, fell down the stairs or had a punch up with someone, that you and your baby would be fine. I now realise that I had been totally misguided here - they don't call them dramatic storylines for nothing! Getting pregnant and staying pregnant, while abstaining from all manner of things from wine to D.I.Y. would still not ensure a problem free pregnancy for me. As a female, it seems we spend half our life trying not to fall pregnant and the other half trying desperately hard to conceive.

My diary is a true account of our journey towards becoming parents, including the highs and the lows along the way. We had a couple of false starts that at the time were heart breaking. I have tried not to dwell on the negative too much but feel it is important to include all that we experienced in this diary. Hopefully everything will go smoothly for you but if things should go wrong, as they did for us, I hope you will find some comfort in reading my experiences and realise you are not alone.

The upside is that through perseverance and a little bit of luck we are now the proud parents of the most adorable baby ever - I am slightly biased of course!

At the end of each week I have included useful tips and information that helped me. Obviously, I am not a doctor and if you are worried about anything you should always seek professional advice. I hope to be your companion as you take a trip along the most amazing road that leads to an even more amazing place that I like to call 'Baby Land'.

Try, try, and try again...

Ok so we have already ascertained that my knowledge of pregnancy could be written on a postage stamp and still have space! As we kept trying and I kept having periods, we realised that this whole pregnancy lark was maybe a bit more complicated than we had anticipated. It was time to educate ourselves and fast. After buying a couple of pregnancy magazines and surfing the net I learnt the following:

- To get pregnant you need to be ovulating (I didn't even know what that was until I read up about it. No wonder I failed Biology at school!) Ovulation usually happens between ten and fourteen days from the first day of your period and you may be able to identify it by a change in vaginal discharge which becomes like egg white in texture. I have had this so many times in my life and never realised why. When I was chatting to a friend she made me feel heaps better by stating that she too had wondered what it was and put it down to an infection. It's good to know I'm not the only uninformed girl out there!

- Ovulation denotes a woman's most fertile time and if you are lucky enough to fall pregnant straight away you may experience a small amount of blood loss called an 'implantation bleed' that you could mistake for a very light period. It is caused by the egg bedding into the wall of your uterus, although not every woman experiences this. One thing I have learned along the way is that every pregnancy is unique and it is best to seek professional advice if you have any unanswered questions. However try not to worry too much if your experience is not following the 'text book'.

Dave and I were married in July and started trying for a baby pretty much straight away. We thought it would be a breeze; neither of us smoked, we didn't drink excessively, and I had been off the contraceptive pill for about fourteen years. We both had healthy diets, me vegan and Dave vegetarian - vegan when I was cooking, and we were both in good shape health-wise. I was teaching dance to adults and children, totalling some twenty hours a week of physical exercise and Dave was a keen runner, frequently taking part in marathons.

We worked out that on our wedding night it would have been practically impossible for me to fall pregnant as my period started the following day, although there are always exceptions to the rule. Once my period was over we tried again and I convinced myself I was pregnant until another period started just fifteen days after the last one - these were such confusing times. The following day my period stopped, that got my hopes up again, only to have them dashed when I had a full-on period some six days later. On a positive note, my disappointment also brought about a realisation that I truly did want a baby and for probably the first time in my life I actually felt ready to be a mum. That was quite a big revelation for me, as previously I had always felt that if I were pregnant I would feel like I had a little alien inside my tummy. It's funny what you learn about yourself as time passes; I had never thought I would get married and up until Dave proposed had never really seen the point of it. How differently I feel now, being married has made us feel even stronger as a couple and becoming parents would be the icing on the cake.

We calculated that the next time I would be fertile landed when Dave was working away - typical! Apparently sperm can stay alive for four days inside a woman and there is a twelve hour window of opportunity when the egg is released. At this point I was seriously beginning to wonder how any woman managed to conceive with such constraints, no wonder they call it the 'miracle of birth'!

We made love on the Monday and Tuesday before Dave went away and on the Friday when he returned, but I didn't feel confident that I'd even ovulated. Now that I knew what to look out for I was more aware and checked every time I went to the loo - not something I would recommend you do as it just drives you nuts!

On the Saturday we went on a camping holiday to the South of France, during which time we had so much nooky that I think Dave thought all his Birthdays and Christmases had come at once. I have since learnt that the quality of semen is not as good if you have too much sex, doh! So it is actually better to have a few days rest, but what can I say we were on a mission. By the Wednesday I thought I may be ovulating so I practically ravished Dave - not that he was putting up too much of a fight, might I add. We drove to Cannes and enjoyed swimming and relaxing on the gorgeous beach there.

On the Friday I experienced some light spotting and guessed that this month it wasn't going to happen for us either. Despite having a wonderful time in Cannes I felt a bit quiet and reflective, not normal emotions for me as I'm usually chatty and up-beat. We drove to the next town on our journey and on the way stopped at those yucky French loos that are just a hole you have to squat over. As I finished my wee, hovering over the hole and trying not to get wet feet as I pulled the flush, I felt really dizzy. I put it down to the heat, the position I had been in, and maybe the fact that that I had been holding my breath as they were not the most pleasantly fragrant of conveniences. Over the next few days I started to feel a little bit different to usual. I didn't exactly have pains anywhere but a slight pulling sensation inside, not unlike the feeling I get when a period is due, but I surely couldn't be due one again so soon, could I?

The rest of our holiday was lovely, it was so good to relax and just enjoy each other's company. We got back home at 2.30 am on Monday morning, were in bed by 3 am and amazingly I was up again by 8 am, while Dave lay lifeless in bed, exhausted no doubt from all the driving. In a couple of hours I had unpacked our cases, done 3 wash loads, baked a malt loaf and tidied up. I was convinced my period was about to start as I always get a bit of a 'nesting' urge around that time.

A few days later when my period still hadn't arrived I bought myself a pregnancy test and with a mix of anticipation and excitement carefully followed all the instructions. After waiting for the test to work Dave and I looked at the results, looked at each other in confusion, and then re-read the instructions! My test stick had a strong, horizontal blue line that on its own meant that

I was not pregnant. But as we looked at the test, a very pale, vertical blue line was appearing, which could mean I was pregnant. The instruction leaflet didn't shed much light, so all in all it was pretty anti-climatic. I was kicking myself for not spending the extra few pounds for a digital test that would have actually said, 'Yes' or 'No'. Dave and I were only laughing about an advert for it on TV recently. It's a clever commercial where right up till the last minute you are not sure what it is for. Just when you think it is about a new car or gadget the male voice-over says, 'It's the most sophisticated bit of technology you will ever pee on!'

In the end we decided to leave it for a couple of days and retest on Friday, which took an age to come around. I had the day off work and we planned to go to Brighton. I took a test before we left and it was pretty much the same as the previous one, maybe a slightly darker blue line - although that might just have been wishful thinking. We went into Boots with my test stick to ask the pharmacist what it meant. The lady I spoke to took one look and said, 'It's fairly conclusive'. When she noted the bewildered looks on our faces she elaborated that, 'Yes', it was a positive test result, and the reason for the pale blue line was possibly that as I was testing so early on that my pregnancy hormones were not high enough to show clearly on the test yet. I found myself clapping my hands in excitement and having a little jump for joy. We stocked up on 9 months supply of vitamins for me to take, it was funny to think that when I'd finished all of the tablets that we would hopefully have a baby. The rest of the day was lovely, especially when we met up with Stephen, our wedding photographer and he gave us all the photos he took back in July. Looking through the pictures I felt a mixture of emotions, nostalgia for the fantastic day of our wedding but also excitement and anticipation for the arrival of a baby in the future.

Before we left Brighton I bought myself a pregnancy magazine that seemed pretty informative as I flicked through it. From what I could glean it would appear that I was probably 4 weeks pregnant, as you counted the days from the first day of your last period. That would make the baby, or embryo as it was medically referred to at this point, between the size of a pin head and a grain of rice. Dave kept asking me how 'pin head' was doing which was really sweet. The magazine also had a week by week guide as to what was going on with your body and it would appear that morning sickness was a couple of weeks off - there's something to look forward to! It also had an informative section on work related benefits that I read up on. I ignored all the articles on pushchairs they had tested, weaning etc, as I didn't want to tempt fate with things that seemed so far away. We both desperately wanted to tell people, especially our family but we decided to wait until we were safely through the first crucial 3 to 4 months. It was going to be difficult keeping my pregnancy a secret at work as it was pretty demanding - what with all the dancing around and especially if I was feeling queasy. Although one good thing about my job was that I started in the afternoon most days, so I might just get away with it.

I went online and typed 'vegan pregnancy' into our search engine. It was important to me to remain vegan but at the same time I didn't want to do anything to compromise the health of our baby. The Vegan Society website was very informative and along with the vitamins I was taking I needed to ensure I ate plenty of the following:

dried beans, lentils, tofu, calcium fortified soya milk, leafy green vegetables, nutritional yeast, flaxseed, flaxseed oil, rapeseed oil, canola oil, walnuts, soya beans, tempeh, bagels and whole grains.

I also ordered a book called 'Pregnancy, children and the vegan diet' by Dr Michael Klaper and 'Vegetarian and Vegan Mother and Baby Guide' by Rose Elliot.

I felt ready to embrace and enjoy every part of this pregnancy. I also decided to keep a weekly record of my weight gain and a food journal, just in case I got a doctor who thought I was a crazy vegan who wasn't getting enough nutrients in my diet. (See the meal planner at the end of the book).

It felt fantastic being pregnant, but so hard not telling anyone - especially at work when I would rather not be jumping up and down all day. I had feelings not unlike period pains - but without the pain if that makes sense. Dave and I had affectionately been referring to the baby as 'rice head' as that was the size my magazine informed me that the embryo would be at 5 weeks. I didn't want to wish the time away but I was keen to get beyond 12 weeks when the chances of miscarriage get lower. Dave tried to tell me not to worry, which I didn't think I was doing excessively but it was hard to ignore the statistics I kept reading about in my magazine.

Dave's brother, Doug, was competing in a triathlon and we went along to support him. Now I have a terrible fear of heights and was not a happy bunny when I saw that we would be required to go over a very high, rickety scaffold bridge to get to the start line. I managed to get a steward to let me cross the road at the beginning of the race but at the end I was confronted by a really mean woman who swore at me when I asked if I could go back the same way. She was so aggressive that I did say to her that I felt her attitude was totally uncalled for. She let us pass but I felt rather shaken and upset. I pulled myself together, but later I felt some unpleasant dragging sensations inside that worried me and made me determined to steer clear of stressful situations in the future.

Apart from that occasion I felt pretty much the same as usual, although my boobs ached in the morning and seemed to be a bit larger, which Dave thought was great!

Tuesday 19th September

I had my first doctor's appointment today which was rather nerve-wracking as I usually avoided the place at all costs. I saw a lovely doctor who took my blood pressure but to my surprise didn't ask me to do a pregnancy test as she said the shop ones were pretty reliable. She told me my 'due date' was the 18th May which was what I had calculated it to be - yay, all the reading was paying off!

I left the surgery with a magazine called 'Emma's Diary' she had given me, an agreement to get a blood test done in the next 7-10 days and a big smile of relief that it had been so straightforward.

My happiness was short-lived, as in the evening during my adult ballet class I started to experience some strange pulling sensations. I nipped to the toilet while my ladies were having a stretch and was upset to see pale pink on the tissue. I wasn't sure if that meant I was about to have a miscarriage but decided not to do the rest of the lesson to be on the safe side. I rang Dave and thankfully he was close by and came straight over to pick me up.

I felt like crying but instead tried to stay calm and just prayed that our baby was OK. When we got home I went on the internet looking for any information I could find. It seemed that pale pink/brown blood loss was fairly common. If it was red and painful that was when it was time to worry. In the end, I decided to take it easy and got an early night, although it was hard to sleep as I lay there worrying I might be losing our baby.

Wednesday 20th September

When I woke at 7.30 am another trip to the toilet confirmed my worse fears as there was more blood loss. I rang the doctors surgery and they advised me to go straight to the hospital. We saw a nurse in A&E who asked me to do a urine sample and then sent me to another part of the hospital where I waited for ages to see a nurse. The entire time I wasn't in any pain I just felt so tearful and incredibly sad. When I was eventually seen, the nurse explained that I would need an internal scan, but that as I was in the early stages of pregnancy they might not be able to detect the baby. She did the scan and as she'd expected where the sac that contained the baby should be didn't show on the scan. Next I had a blood test to ascertain what levels of pregnancy hormones I had, if they were high then the pregnancy might still be viable. It wasn't too bad; I just didn't look as she put the needle in my arm. The nurse said that I could go home and they would ring me with the results in a few hours.

Dave had got a job in Scotland, of all places, starting today for the best part of a week. I really didn't want to be on my own, but I also didn't want him to feel bad for going or to be worrying about me, so I put on a brave face until he left then bawled my eyes out for the rest of the day. I got to a stage when I didn't think I could have any liquid left in me as I had been crying for so long. I was also in the tricky situation of not knowing what to tell my work place. When we got married earlier in the year my boss didn't speak to me for 3 days and when she finally did it was to say, 'Don't you dare get pregnant!' I'm still not sure whether she was joking or not so I had mixed feelings about what to tell her.

I rang my friend Wendy in the end, as she always seems to be able to put things into perspective - she's a professional counsellor so I shouldn't be surprised. Her thoughts were that there are some things in life you have no control over but other things you do. So while I couldn't prevent myself from losing our baby, I could take control over my work situation and choose whether or not to go in and what to say to them. She also said such a lovely thing to me which was; that she had never met a couple more in love, content and supportive of each other than Dave and I, and that when it was meant to happen we would create a wonderful child together.

I came off the phone feeling a bit better and after speaking to Dave we both decided that I wasn't going to elaborate on things at work, after all it really was none of their business. The rest of the evening dragged by with nothing to do except feel sorry for myself. I was missing Dave so much, but tried to hold it together when I spoke to him on the phone as he had a job to do and I didn't want to make things harder for him.

Thursday 21st September

I woke up crying, which was not the best way to start the day! I couldn't think of a time when I had ever felt so lonely. I was desperate for a hug from Dave; I thought I would cope so much better if he was with me. It was a beautiful sunny day and I wished I could click my fingers and be magically transported to Brighton as I knew that would lift my spirits. I wasn't in pain, I just felt like I was having a really heavy period, but I didn't think I had the strength to make the trip as it was the best part of 2 hours away on the train. I also felt a bit in limbo as I had to return to the hospital the following day for another blood test to check the pregnancy hormone levels to see if they had dropped. In my heart I already knew the answer - the baby had gone - I just didn't feel pregnant anymore, my boobs felt back to normal and when I weighed myself I was 3 pounds lighter than before - although that could just have been from all the tears I had shed!

I decided to text my lovely friend Karen on the off-chance that she might not be busy. She rang me back and I ended up telling her everything. She said she would finish the work she was doing and come over to me as soon as she could. I felt so relieved to have spoken to her and glad I wouldn't be on my own much longer as I didn't want to wallow in sadness anymore.

Karen arrived in the evening and I managed not to cry at all - which was a major achievement for me.

Friday 22nd September

Karen drove me to the hospital for my blood test - this time not in the baby clinic, which was a good thing. In fact it felt a bit like being in Argos as I sat watching the screen for my number to come up. After a wait of 45 minutes I had the test taken by a lovely nurse who was so sympathetic. She had 4 miscarriages herself before having 2 healthy children, so I felt there was still hope for me.

When we got home we spent the rest of the day chatting and looking through mine and Dave's wedding photos.

Saturday 23rd September

Karen sensing my desire to get out the house and clear my head offered to drive us to Brighton for the day. It was beautiful weather and despite numerous toilet stops I had a lovely day. We didn't walk too far, just to The Pavilion, where Dave and I were married and then had lunch sat on the beach. Karen was some time on the phone discussing work with a colleague and I took the opportunity for some quiet time to reflect on things. I threw some pebbles into the sea, some for family and friends and a special one for our baby. Then I threw handfuls into the water with force, a bit like I was throwing my anger and disappointment away. I felt much better afterwards!

Some 7 months had passed since my miscarriage. Dave and I wanted to try for a baby again and after waiting for a 'normal period' we started. I began to feel that all I was thinking about was making a baby and while we had lots of fun practicing I didn't want to become obsessed with it. So with that in mind we found ourselves a distraction in the form of property hunting. We had offers accepted on 2 properties: a 1 bed, investment flat in Folkestone and a 3 bed house in Dover we planned on renovating and selling on. I took on the crazy task of arranging all the mortgages myself, 2 new ones and 2 remortgages. I must have been mad as rather than being less stressful than using a financial advisor it was far worse and incredibly time consuming. It did however take our minds off babies and we just continued trying but without giving it too much thought.

In January I got my hopes up that I might be pregnant again as I had some light spotting just 14 days after my period and I thought it could be an implantation bleed. I was disappointed when the bleeding didn't stop though and turned into a proper period.

Dave and I cracked on with getting our home in London spruced up to let, as we planned to move into the property in Folkestone while Dave renovated the house in Dover. I arranged with friends (who lived near to my work place) to stay with them Monday through to Thursday and the plan was to catch a train to Folkestone after work every Friday to be with Dave for the weekends. The only worry I had was asking my boss if I could swap my days around as I had previously always worked on a Saturday. I plucked up the courage to ask her and the first thing she said was, 'It could have been worse; you could have been telling me you were pregnant!'

I bought essential oils that were reputedly good for fertility and tried not to get stressed out while I waited for my boss to get back to me with her decision about my hours. Time passed and before I knew it half-term was upon me and with it the chaotic week it entailed, as the children I taught came for an entire week of 'drama, song and dance'. We also had builders in working on the roof; they made lots of mess and noise and worse still they were using particularly smelly chemicals.

By the end of the week I was wiped out and glad that it was Friday at last. Dave had made us a delicious meal, after which I went to bed and slept for 12 hours!

After a relaxing weekend I was due to have a meeting at work with a lady from head office regarding my request for swapping my days around. I felt quite hyper all morning and on a whim decided to take a pregnancy test before I went in. To my total delight it was positive! Although I was over the moon, my happiness was tinged with apprehension after what happened last time. It did, however, explain why I had felt strange recently and my mega long sleep.

My meeting went well with head office and I got my new hours approved. I did also tell the lady that I was pregnant and didn't feel able to tell my boss. She said that it was up to me, but in her opinion it would be better to mention it as I had concerns regarding the building works that could be addressed if I explained my situation. She said that my boss would be able to arrange a risk assessment of my work place that would reassure me that there were no dangers to our baby.

I had the following week off as annual leave during which Dave and I moved into our property in Folkestone. I most definitely was feeling pregnant and my sense of smell had gone into over-drive, I felt especially nauseous when the smell of someone else's fish supper wafted into our bedroom...Yuk!

Back at work the fumes from the roofers' chemicals made me feel light-headed prompting me to tell my boss of my pregnancy. She was pretty good considering she was always telling me not to get pregnant and suggested I took another week's annual leave to give her chance to get the place checked out.

It was a relief to be off work and taking it easy, although I spent most of my week alone as Dave was busy getting stuck into renovating the Dover property. I had read in my pregnancy magazine about lead in old paint etc and decided it was best to avoid being there; instead I took lots of lovely walks along the Leas in Folkestone.

As the time progressed and I got beyond the first 6 weeks (that was when I lost our first baby) I began to feel a bit more confident. I started reading a lovely book by Jools Oliver about her pregnancies called 'Minus Nine to One' and even found myself talking to our baby. My boobs felt enormous and I had 'evening sickness'. I wasn't actually sick but most evenings I felt a bit queasy. Strangely enough I was happy to be experiencing all of these things as it reassured me that my pregnancy was progressing well. One evening I had terrible indigestion and the following afternoon period type pains. I found it difficult to know whether these were normal pregnancy symptoms. I then had a week where I just didn't feel pregnant and slept badly each night with lots on my mind. I woke one morning with what I could only describe as a pain in my heart. I didn't think I was particularly stressed out, so I tried not to dwell on it and just got on with the things I needed to do around the flat. Apart from that I felt absolutely fine and as I was fast approaching 12 weeks of pregnancy I started to relax and look forward to my first scan.

Wednesday 11th April

Today was a total nightmare at work, the roofers were still working on the building and at one point it sounded as though they all had a power tool switched on full blast. What with that to contend with plus 20 children all running around; it was pretty stressful. When I got home I took a bath and was shocked to see the tell-tale sign once again of pink on the toilet tissue. I tried to stay calm and convince myself that I wasn't having a repeat of last September's experience. My next door neighbour popped in, and on seeing my distress sent his wife around to sit with me while I waited for Dave to come home. I knew that there was nothing that could be done until the morning when I could hopefully get an appointment at the Early Pregnancy Unit (EPU) in the hospital for a scan, so we just had to wait it out.

Thursday 12th April

I tried to get an appointment at the EPU but didn't have any luck so instead Dave drove me to my doctors surgery. It turned out that since my last miscarriage they had changed the rules and you had to be referred by a doctor to get a scan. I had no option but to go to A&E where I was seen by a lovely nurse who said she would make sure I got a scan as soon as possible. Upstairs in the EPU I received the news I had been dreading, that although I was in theory 12 weeks into my pregnancy the baby had stopped developing at about 6 weeks. The nurse explained that I had 3 options: I could go home and let the miscarriage happen naturally, have some tablets to speed it along, or have a procedure known as D&C. I decided to go home and let nature take its course.

By the time we had driven from London to Folkestone we were starving as we had only eaten a banana each all day. We had a pizza and settled down for the night; at this point I wasn't losing much blood. Physically I felt fine just terribly sad.

Friday 13th April

I woke at 2 am in a pool of blood, went to the bathroom and nearly passed out, which wasn't good. I managed to ring NHS Direct and they told me to go to hospital as soon as possible. At the A&E department of Ashford hospital I was seen by a couple of different nurses and had blood taken. They were so kind and sympathetic, one of them held my hand as she explained that my uterus was not acknowledging that the pregnancy was over, hence all the blood loss. She said that she would try to remove as much as possible but that if I kept on bleeding I might have to go to theatre. She then said they would leave Dave and me alone for 5 minutes. Now at this point I seriously thought she was implying that I needed to say goodbye to Dave in case I died! I felt absolutely terrible. In an instant flash I thought about my family and friends, but mostly of Dave and how much I didn't want to leave him. By the time the nurses returned I was inconsolable, which surprised them as I had been fine when they left. Between sobs I told them I didn't want to die, they looked slightly bemused and assured me I wasn't going to die. What a relief! I must be the only person ever to have a near death experience without actually being near death.

Poor Dave, the day had really taken its toll on him. I heard the nurse asking, 'Are you OK?' and assumed she was talking to me. When I looked up I saw Dave's face had drained of colour and he looked like he was going to faint - what a right pair we are! After being given an injection to help contract my uterus I was told I would need to be admitted for the night. I was feeling scared as I was wheeled off on a trolley, I am the worlds worst in hospitals so it was good that Dave was with me. Later he had to leave to drive to Dover to pay our plasterers and I was left alone in a ward with 3 other empty beds. The nurses were all very kind but I kept experiencing such waves of sadness washing over me all day. In the evening

Dave returned with food, magazines and a lovely card for me. He stayed as long as visiting hours permitted, and then I was alone again for the night. After he left I shed a few tears; he rang when he got home to say he had told his mum and she had been fantastic. Although she was sad for us, she was over the moon to hear we had started trying for a family. I still felt terrible as I hated spreading bad news and for weeks I had been visualising giving her and Tony and my mum and dad a copy of the scan of our baby.

Saturday 14th April

In the morning I was seen by a lovely doctor who crouched by the side of my bed, held my hand and was very sympathetic. He said that there was no reason why the next time we tried that Dave and I wouldn't be successful and offered us some counselling as well. While I waited for Dave to come and pick me up I chatted to a really nice girl in the bed opposite and her mum, who encountered many difficulties when she was trying for a family. She had 4 miscarriages, a still birth and a cot death between the births of her 2 daughters. What an inspiration she was. I don't think I would have had the strength to keep trying in the face of so much adversity. I felt better for talking to her as she seemed to understand just how I was feeling. I was discharged from the hospital and told to return on Friday for another scan to make sure everything had gone.

Dave picked me up at 12.30 pm; outside it was a baking hot day and I felt like a prisoner who had just been freed from jail.

We walked to the beach and talked like we never had before. We discussed everything that had happened and the possibility of adopting a child if we couldn't have any of our own. One thing I have learned is that Dave is such a rock to me, this whole experience seemed to have brought us even closer to each other. We both felt so sad to have lost another baby but glad to be alive and together. Later I rang my mum and told her everything; she was absolutely brilliant as was my dad. I realised that we had handled everything all wrong with both miscarriages. Where we hadn't wanted to share sad news we'd bottled everything up between ourselves and as a result felt really alone. All our family and friends were so kind and supportive to us.

It was about 5 weeks before I felt physically and emotionally ready to start trying for a baby again. Dave was busy working on the property in Dover and I was still staying with friends during the week and taking the long train journey at the weekends to see him. It wasn't an ideal situation but we just tried to make the best of it and hoped it wouldn't be for much longer. The months passed and the friends I was living with discovered that they were expecting a baby. I was so pleased for them, but disappointed that it still hadn't happened for us.

In August we had a fantastic camping holiday in France that really lifted our spirits. It was back to reality with a bump however, when we returned to our flat in Folkestone to discover we had been flooded and part of the bedroom ceiling was on the bed. We looked on the bright side, after all it could have been worse, we may well have been in the bed as well! While we waited for the insurance claim to go through we found ourselves 'camping' in the living room on our inflatable mattress from our vacation.

By October I was beginning to give up hope that I would ever fall pregnant after yet another period came and went. Every month I had the same little routine of not drinking alcohol or doing any painting until my period arrived. When it did I promptly got the wine out and helped Dave with the never-ending property renovations that needed doing. We were also still sleeping on our trusty blow-up bed as our managing agents hadn't repaired the ceiling so everything was slightly make-shift to say the least.

Another period comes along...

Wednesday 17th October

It was such a busy day at work with the endless preparations for our Christmas productions - every year I vowed it would be my last and yet here I was again slaving away!

Disappointingly my period started, although I was so stressed out that it was probably a good thing. At least I would be able to help Dave with varnishing the floors in Dover at the weekend. I was beginning to think I would never get pregnant, which was really sad. I busied myself at work, all 10 hours of it, and was absolutely exhausted by the time I finished.

Friday 19th October

I was up at 8 am and at work for 9 am which was a shock to the system, especially after all the extra hours I had put in this week. I spent ages going through the performance schedule, which needed major jiggling around. A couple of my private one-to-one classes had cancelled, which gave me a bit of a break. By the time I got on the train to Folkestone I felt more tired than usual, plus I had hunger/period pains as well. The train was packed and the journey felt arduously long, I was so glad to see Dave when I finally got out of the station and he was waiting to pick me up. We had a lovely meal in the local Chinese restaurant - the staff always joke when we go there that they need to get in extra tofu for us! Once fed and watered I gradually felt my stresses melt away.

Sunday 21st October

Dave and I put a full day in at the house in Dover. We sanded the floors downstairs and then swept thoroughly before varnishing. Dave had a bit of an accident when he knocked the container over and about a pint of varnish spilled across the floor. We quickly tried to spread it as best we could and then varnished ourselves out of the house.

Later back at the flat it was my turn to have an accident when I somehow managed to put curry powder instead of cinnamon into the apple crumble. Luckily I smelt my error before it got as far as the oven - or indeed our mouths - and started again.

Monday 22nd October

Today was a really full-on day; we sanded and varnished the floors again in Dover before returning to Folkestone for lunch. By early evening we were in Brighton as we needed to check on the damage to the ceiling of our flat there that had been flooded a while back (what is it with us and water?) In the morning we were getting a quote from a builder to have it fixed, which should hopefully be covered on our insurance. We spent the rest of the evening going through boxes in the loft and adding things we had brought with us. Dave also scraped the adhesive off some tiles that had come loose in the bathroom, ready to re-stick. We both wanted to be living in Brighton, but realised we would have to be patient and wait until we had Dover and Folkestone sorted out - oh the joys of property developing!

Tuesday 23rd October

We met the builder and he seemed decent enough - no horse tied up outside!

It was such a lovely day that after breakfast at a great veggie cafe we walked to the beach.

Refreshed from a dose of sea-air we returned to the flat. Dave glued the bathroom tiles back up, although if we did end up moving here they seriously needed to go as they were champagne with sprigs of flowers on them. Lovely, not!

I went for a wander around The Lanes and bought a couple of Christmas presents. We finally got back to Folkestone at 9 pm.

Tips & things to do

- Well, strictly speaking you haven't even conceived your baby and yet this week is still referred to as 'week one' of your pregnancy. This week you are actually having the last period you can expect for quite some time. Note down the date your period starts as your doctor will want to know. The first day of your last period is when you start counting the weeks from.

- If you haven't done so already now is a good time to have a think about your lifestyle and diet, are there any changes you want to make? Such as giving up smoking or drinking alcohol, taking more exercise or improving your diet.

- Make sure you are taking a good folic acid supplement. Folic acid is vital to help your baby's brain develop properly and helps prevent neural tube defects such as spina bifida. In addition to taking supplements, there are foods that are naturally rich in folic acid - broccoli, green leafy vegetables and brussel sprouts. As well as yoghurt, milk and yeast rich products like Marmite. (Sprouts and Marmite that's two things you will either love to eat or detest).

- In addition to eating a healthy, well-balanced diet it's a good idea to take some vitamin supplements. I took some great ones called 'Pregnacare' from Boots that were specially formulated to be taken during pregnancy, through to breastfeeding and beyond.

D.I.Y. Diva...

Wednesday 24th October

We went back to Dover to do the last coat of varnish after sanding it all down again. It was time-consuming but looked absolutely fantastic, even if I say so myself. We ordered a kitchen from Howdens that should get delivered tomorrow. We also ended up buying another inflatable mattress as ours kept going down, probably from all the nooky we were having.

I felt so tired today which was hardly surprising after all the driving and D.I.Y. recently.

Thursday 25th October

I started to experience some strange pains and dragging sensations which were a bit of a worry. A pharmacist in Sainsbury's recommended that I got it checked out at a local hospital in Folkestone. I was seen by a lovely lady who checked that I didn't have a urine infection. In her opinion she thought my pains might be psychological, as our baby would have been born this week. Later on, as I was channel hopping on TV, I caught a bit of a sex education programme talking about Chlamydia and other horrible diseases. I am such a hypochondriac that

I soon had myself very stressed out and convinced I had something like that.

Friday 26th October
I decided to try and be positive instead of tormenting myself with worrying about things I couldn't do anything about - easier said than done!

I booked myself a Reiki treatment for following week, as in the past I had found my body responded well to the healing; also it was something to look forward to.

Dave and I ended up taking some of the cupboards back to Howdens as they had delivered the wrong ones; we also returned some plinth we didn't need.

I telephoned my boss to ask her if I could take next week off sick as although I didn't feel ill I just wanted to take some time to sort my body out. She was fine about it. I was so relieved and happy that I would have another week with Dave; hopefully my pains would disappear too.

Tuesday 30th October
The last couple of days I had been incredibly tired and was half tempted to stay in bed today. I did an ovulation test, as we had been busy at the baby-making practice, but it malfunctioned. I decided there wasn't much point in trying another test as my body was still playing up with the odd dragging sensation and twinge of pain.

Tips & things to do
- If you want to increase your chances of conceiving then you could look into purchasing a home ovulation kit. The one I bought was pretty simple to use, if you were ovulating a smiley face came up on

the stick after you had taken a wee on it, indicating it was a great time to grab your partner for some baby-making practice.

- You could start a pregnancy diary or journal; it doesn't need to be elaborate. Keep a record of important changes you are experiencing, from pregnancy symptoms to weight gain and cravings for example.

- Once your period finishes your body will produce hormones that will ripen the egg that will become your baby. Depending on the length of your menstrual cycle the end of this week may be a good time to try for a baby... Good Luck!

Amazing Reiki...

Thursday 1st November

Dave drove me to Canterbury for my Reiki treatment in the afternoon. Amazingly without me even saying what my problem was the practitioner, a lovely lady called Cheryl, went straight to my pelvic area and said she felt lots of activity there. I told her about my miscarriages and she said she could sense the shock from them still there in my body and that my head was full of stuff - no surprises there! I ended up getting quite tearful and emotional but it was great to talk and get things off my chest. The treatment was so relaxing and I booked another session for Saturday.

Friday 2nd November

We had a nice morning spent making love and just chilling out.

Later we cleared the bedrooms at Dover as they were getting carpeted the next day, yippee! I touched up the paintwork on the skirting boards that had got scuffed and hoped they wouldn't dry out too patchy. I realised that I had spent most of the day without experiencing any of my dodgy pains which was amazing, maybe the Reiki had helped.

Saturday 3rd November

I had another brilliant session with Cheryl today; she did a mixture of Reiki and Aura Soma on me. I hadn't come across that particular therapy before but found it was really great. She had lots of bottles filled with liquid of every colour imaginable; many of them were dual colours that looked so beautiful and jewel-like. Cheryl asked me to select 4 different bottles choosing those I felt most drawn to, and then she explained what my choices meant. Interestingly it came up that I should be expressing myself through writing. I felt remarkably relaxed and happy for the rest the day and in the evening Dave and I watched a great firework display.

Sunday 4th November

It was such a beautiful day today and I was feeling so much better. All my niggling little pains had gone and I was struggling to remember what they felt like.

Dave and I had a wonderful time together; we walked all the way along the beach from Folkestone to Sandgate, then back to Folkestone harbour. We chatted about so many things and started making little plans for when we finally moved to Brighton.

In the afternoon we drove to Howletts Animal Park where we had a fabulous time. We got up close to elephants, monkeys, tigers and lemurs and I loved every minute of it, what a perfect day.

Monday 5th November

I thought my boss was expecting me back at work today but it turned out she had covered my classes until tomorrow so I felt like I had a reprieve.

Dave and I wallpapered the kitchen in Dover and on our way back to Folkestone fed the ducks at the park. Once at the flat I cooked an amazing veggie shepherd's pie and apple crumble, then we snuggled up together.

Tuesday 6th November

Dave left early to get to Dover to see how the carpet was coming along. I chilled out in the flat, watched our wedding DVD and had a relaxing bath. I wasn't looking forward to returning to work and left as late as possible - going the scenic route to the station via the seafront. As I sat on the train I felt the horrible pains come back again. I could see I was going to have to work hard at staying relaxed and positive.

This proved harder than expected; as soon as I got to work I noticed I had been given an extra class to teach and the receptionist had put a 4 year old child in a class I taught for 5-8 year olds. I did find myself slamming the office door in annoyance.

Tips & things to do

- This is the week you will most likely conceive your baby, although you will probably be blissfully unaware of it. As your egg travels down your fallopian tube the sperm swim towards it. When the egg and sperm meet the amazing new life starts.

- Whether you have been trying for a baby for years, months or weeks make it the relaxing, enjoyable and intimate moment it deserves to be. If you have been trying to conceive for a long time you may find that the act of making love has become more of a task or mission with a baby being your prize. This week rekindle the romance with your partner and concentrate on just being with each other.

- Try to take time to relax. I found my Reiki sessions were a fantastic opportunity for me to switch off from all the stresses of everyday life. You may prefer to try some relaxation exercises such as meditation or yoga, or simply take some time out to do whatever suits you.

To resign or not to resign, that is the question?

Thursday 8th November

I had an appointment to get checked out at the doctor's today and was seen by a really unsympathetic doctor. When I told her all the symptoms I had experienced recently she said, 'What do you want me to do about it?' I bit my tongue, tried not to cry and politely asked for a Chlamydia test and a cervical smear just to be on the safe side. Both the tests were uncomfortable but at least they were done now. When I told her what the nurse in Folkestone had told me, she said words to the effect that people would make up all types of stories to explain the unexplainable. She was such hard work; maybe I got her on a bad day.

Saturday 10th November

I was back in Folkestone with Dave again for the weekend, hooray! I went for another Reiki treatment, which was brilliant. I felt so much more myself; Dave had noticed the change in me and was pleased I was back to my jolly old self again.

I made the momentous decision to hand in my notice at work - even though I had been there for 7 years and didn't actually have another job lined up. My resignation had been prompted by a combination of things, mostly the fact that I missed Dave so much and found it just too hard only seeing him at weekends. The friends I had been living with in London said they needed to reclaim my room ready for when their baby arrived and since I had been back at work my boss had been tying to increase my hours, but not my pay! Dave and I talked it through and I thought it was the best decision I'd made in ages, I already felt a huge weight lifted off my shoulders. We spent the evening typing up my resignation letter.

Monday 12th November

We woke at 9 am and had a relaxing morning together, although I kept getting butterflies at the thought of handing in my resignation. In the end I typed up two differently dated letters, one for today and one for next week. I still felt like there was so much up in the air, I was waiting for the test results to come back from the doctor's which might affect my decision. Also to keep my options open I had run the possibility of staying just 2 nights a week at my friend's house past them as well.

As I sat on the train with the letters practically burning a hole in my bag I decided that I was going to go through with resigning today. Sometimes in life you have to just take a leap of faith and hope for the best. The thought of continuing as I had been indefinitely was not how I wanted to live my life and with everything being so difficult it felt as if I was being pushed into making this decision anyway.

As she read my letter, the expression on my bosses face was priceless. Amazingly she had not seen it coming at all, which surprised me as I thought that my unhappiness must have been apparent to everyone - maybe I was a better actress than I thought! She didn't try to persuade me to stay and there were no sweeping gestures of a huge pay rise or less hours to tempt me, so she really did make it quite easy for me.

Later though it was a lot harder telling my customers, some of whom I'd become good friends with. A couple of my little girls I taught tap dancing to started to cry when I told them which really tugged on my heart strings.

Tips & things to do

- This week you may experience some light spotting that you could mistake for a period; however it is more likely the implantation bleed. Not every woman gets this light spotting, I didn't, so you will just have to wait and see!

- Take time to talk with your partner regarding how you both feel about becoming parents; are there any aspects of your lives you would like to change?

I'm pregnant!

Wednesday 14th November

I had been planning on telling my 50-plus tap class (where in fact the average age was 78!) the news of my leaving. But as I gathered them around, I had scarcely opened my mouth when one of them totally jumped the gun crying out, 'I knew it, you're pregnant!' Without engaging my brain first I found myself biting back, that no, I wasn't pregnant, that I had in fact lost 2 babies, that I was totally unhappy being separated from Dave and that I had handed in my notice. Whoops that really didn't go as planned! Several of the ladies I had known for ages were upset that I was leaving but were very supportive of my decision.

It was a pretty emotional day all round, I kind of wished I could just slip away without having to tell anyone else as it was just so hard. I started packing away the costumes I had lent to children over the years into my big trunks from boarding school and that set me off crying again as it felt like the end of an era.

Friday 16th November

I had a bit of a lie-in today, I kept expecting my period to start as today was 26 days and that was a long cycle for me. I had a stomach ache last night so I was sure it was on its way, although part of me was worrying that maybe I was pregnant. I know that seems crazy as I had been wishing for it to happen for ages but I thought having those horrible tests and the stress recently would not make it ideal. I decided to buy a test to take at the weekend if my period hadn't started by then.

Sunday 18th November

I woke up with a really sore throat and decided to take a pregnancy test as my period had still not arrived. To my shock it was positive. How on earth was that possible and why of all months this one? I was pleased but the timing was bad, especially as I had been pretty stressed out recently. If I'd known I was pregnant I wouldn't have had the smear test done, drank wine or varnished the floors in Dover and I certainly wouldn't have spent the last week clearing out the filthiest of rooms at work either! I wasn't sure whether to complete my last 2 weeks of work or ask if I could leave immediately.

Monday 19th November

I still had a sore throat and was feeling tired and a bit emotional. As I made the long train journey from Folkestone into work I was already missing Dave. I felt quite subdued as I wanted to be excited to be pregnant but I was scared in case it went wrong again, also I didn't even feel pregnant.

Work was hard, when I told my 7 year olds, who I taught ballet to, that I was leaving, a couple of them cried, which made me feel so bad.

Tuesday 20th November

I managed to get a doctor's appointment before work today and was seen by a lovely nurse who said she would ensure I got an early scan. At least then I would know if there was a heartbeat and wouldn't feel quite so in limbo.

A lady from Head Office rang me to say that I didn't have to honour working for the last 2 weeks of my notice and that I would still get paid. I decided to take her up on her offer and spent the rest of the evening saying my good-byes to customers.

Tips & things to do

- You will probably have noticed by now that your period is late and if you take a test it may well show up positive.

- You might be feeling out-of-sorts, stressed out, tearful and moody to name just a few - it's those pesky hormones kicking in! Physically your boobs could be sore, you may feel really tired or even a bit sick already.

- Book an appointment to see your doctor; he or she will calculate your 'due date' for you, take your blood pressure and answer any questions you may have at this stage.

- To calculate your 'due date' for yourself. Take the first day of your last period, add on a year, take three months off, and finally add one week back on. Confused? Don't worry it's only a guess anyway, babies come when they're ready.

- If you have had any miscarriages in the past ask your doctor if you can have an appointment for an early scan.

- If, like me, you did things early on in your pregnancy that were not ideal then try not to beat yourself up about it. One thing I have learnt is that babies are resilient little things. If your pregnancy is meant to be it will be and anyway you can't undo what's been done so don't stress yourself out about it too much. If you are worried about anything ask your doctor. Believe me they are used to being asked all sorts of random questions by mums-to-be.

Feeling like death on a dish...

Wednesday 21st November

My last day at work and my 50-plus tap dancing class had done a whip round and gave me a card and some M&S vouchers. It was emotional saying goodbye to them all as they are such lovely ladies, but I took their addresses and promised to let them know how I was doing. Some of the girls I taught also gave me a lovely bouquet of flowers, bless them. As I left I was sad but felt a sense of relief as well that this time I was going to give this pregnancy the best chance I could of going the distance.

Thursday 22nd November

I spent the entire morning lying on the couch at my friend's house trying to psyche myself up to leave to catch the train home to Folkestone. I waited ages for a bus, laden with bags and nearly gave up. I did eventually catch the train and spent the whole journey with my head against the window dozing. Dave picked me up from the station; neither of us could quite believe that I'd given up my job and that after next weekend I wouldn't be returning to London. I was so glad to be with him, even though I felt like death on a dish!

Saturday 24th November

I stayed in bed all day yesterday and today - well, when I say bed I mean our inflatable mattress - as we still didn't have a proper bed. The insurance had gone through for it, but there didn't seem much point buying one until the ceiling had been fixed, which was taking an age to get sorted out. Our managing agents really do take the 'manage' out of managing!

My throat felt much better today but the lurgy had spread to my head which felt like it was in a vice. Every time I got up to go to the bathroom each step I took hurt it. I was so grateful not to be slogging away at work still. When Dave got home from another hard days graft on the house in Dover, he cooked us a delicious veggie shepherd's pie - that was just what I needed.

Sunday 25th November

I felt heaps better today, so I ventured out of the flat for some fresh air walking along the seafront. I stopped off at WHSmith and bought a pregnancy book to read up on. Dave was working all day and I managed to remain upright for most of it which was quite an achievement for me.

Later on I rang my mum and dad and told them I was pregnant. They were both extremely pleased for us - let's hope it is a case of 3rd time lucky!

Tips & things to do

- If you haven't done so already, treat yourself to a pregnancy book or magazine. If you are anything like me you will probably have a million questions needing answering. My pregnancy bible was

'Expecting, Everything you need to know about pregnancy labour and birth' by Anna McGrail and Daphne Metland.

- If you are feeling run-down or poorly - as I was - then just roll with it. If you are able to take some sick leave from work then do. There is so much happening to your body right now, so try not to be too hard on yourself.

- I became addicted to magazines that told me the size of my baby each week. Your baby or 'embryo' as it is referred to at this stage is the size of a grain of rice.

- You may notice your sense of smell has increased making certain things really stomach turning. I also found I needed the loo more often, especially at night.

- Your boobs may be feeling tender and larger than usual.

- Many couples decide to wait until they have reached the 'safer' 12 week mark before telling family or friends of their pregnancy. However, it's a personal choice - we felt we needed the extra support earlier on, in case things went wrong again.

'How do you spell squirrel?'

Thursday 29th November

We pottered around in the morning, doing all the filing that had built up in my absence. We drove to London to stay with our friends Emma and Al for the night, as I had a scan first thing in the morning and was still registered with the doctors there. We had a lovely meal and ended up going to bed later than we planned - just as well because I found it hard to get off to sleep with thoughts running through my head.

Friday 30th November

I slept badly last night, worrying about the prospect of having a scan to see if I was still pregnant.

Dave and I were up and out early to be at the hospital for 8.50 am. We waited ages to be seen and I hated being there again as it just reminded me of our previous two visits. I had convinced myself that this baby would not survive either so I was totally surprised when the screen revealed a tiny little blob, complete with a heartbeat! We both ended up in tears, of joy this time, and once we were in the car we started texting our family to let them know the good news.

Saturday 1st December

Dave and I were having a wonderful morning in the park feeding the squirrels until one bit me. Typically it wasn't just a friendly nip, the little critter drew blood. I went from thinking how cute squirrels are to remembering all the times people have said to me that squirrels are just rats with good PR!

Dave took me to hospital - goodness me I've spent an awful lot of time in A&E recently - to get checked out. By the time I got to the reception area I was convinced I was going to be diagnosed with rabies or something similar. The girl behind the desk looked at me in surprise when I told her what had happened then asked, 'How do you spell squirrel?' I was seen by a nice male nurse who wasn't able to find out if my tetanus shot was up to date and explained that even if it was due there wasn't much they could do for me as they don't give boosters if you're pregnant. I spent the rest of the day hoping I wouldn't start foaming at the mouth!

In the evening we went to watch my work place Christmas production at a local theatre. It was so strange - not to mention civilised - to watch it front of house from a comfy chair for a change. The last few years I was usually to be found backstage running around like a headless chicken. At the end of the show I was presented with some flowers and £40 of John Lewis vouchers, nice but not much to show for 7 years of hard work!

Sunday 2nd December

We returned to the theatre for the matinee of a ballet production. Once again I was in the novel position of watching, while the rest of the staff ran around dressing children, applying make-up and taking toilet break duties.

I hadn't done any of the choreography or costumes for this show so I was able to sit back and relax not worrying, as I usually do, if little Vikki would make her quick change or not.

As with so many things my final goodbye was anti-climatic - Dave and I slipped away, unnoticed - while the remaining staff wrestled with putting costumes away, reuniting children with their parents and the million and one other things that needed doing to restore the theatre back to its original state.

We drove back to our friend's house to pick up my belongings and said our goodbyes. Once on the road, Dave and I chatted about the shows, my work and the fact that I was leaving all that and London behind. I felt the most wonderful sense of freedom wash over me, just extremely glad to be with Dave and our tiny baby - ready to start afresh.

Tips & things to do

- If you have an early scan you will be lucky enough to meet your baby for the first time - albeit that all you will see is a tiny blob about the size of a pea!

- I know I most certainly didn't practice what I preach, but try to reassess your life and make any changes that will ensure it is as free from stress as possible. Avoid vicious squirrels!

- If you have never taken regular exercise then don't jump into starting any strenuous new exercise regimes. Gentle walking, yoga and swimming are all great ways to keep fit throughout your pregnancy.

- Surf the net for information on pregnancy, one of my favourite sites www.babycentre.co.uk gives you a weekly update on how your baby is developing as well as the changes you can expect your body to be going through. BabyCentre gives advice from preconception, pregnancy and birth right up to your baby's 5th birthday.

- When you have your first doctor's appointment he or she will give you a pregnancy pack that usually contains a great little magazine called 'Emma's Diary'. You may also get a leaflet to take to your nearest pharmacist to claim your free 'Bounty Pack' full of money-off vouchers and samples relating to you and your baby.

- If you have any worries or concerns always seek medical advice. If you can't reach your doctor then NHS Direct is really useful.

Sleeping for my country...

Thursday 6th December

I was relishing every moment of not being at work and had enjoyed my week so far. Dave played our wedding and honeymoon DVD - that had me crying, but in a good way. I unpacked my belongings and at last I started to feel at home. It was hard to believe that for the last 7 months I had been living out of a suitcase. I had hardly any personal belongings with me during the week when I was staying with friends and all the rest of my treasures had been boxed up at the flat in Folkestone. It was so nice to arrange some photos on my bedside drawers and to be reunited with all my clothes again. I wasn't sure whether it was from all the unpacking or because I was pregnant but I felt absolutely exhausted.

Sunday 9th December

The house in Dover finally turned a corner and was nearly finished - just 5 months later than we had originally planned! We hoped to move into it soon as the flat in Folkestone was driving us nuts; between the useless managing agents who still hadn't fixed our bedroom ceiling and a noisy neighbour above us who left her

TV on full blast all night long. The only thing that had been holding things up was that the central heating in Dover had packed in, but today Dave got it working again, hooray!

I spent the day feeling decidedly icky. I wasn't actually sick but felt queasy and had to keep lying down. In the evening the top of my right leg was really aching with an unpleasant dragging sensation that was only relieved when Dave gave me a massage, bless him.

Tuesday 11th December

Although I had been feeling incredibly tired recently, I found the energy to do some Christmas shopping today. Dave and I drove to Brighton where we picked out some great gifts for family and friends, then finished the day with a lovely meal in our favourite veggie restaurant, Terre à Terre.

Tips & things to do

- Listen to your body - if you're tired then rest; try to get as much sleep in now as possible. If you're not working then an afternoon nap is great for boosting your dwindling energy supplies.

- In one of my magazines as well as telling me the size of my baby each week it also told me the size of my uterus. So this week my baby was the size of a bean and my uterus a small orange - I wonder why they compare everything to food?

- As your uterus grows you could experience cramp-like pains and twinges. If you are at all concerned speak to your doctor.

- Talking of food - make sure that your diet is full of lots of healthy things. Even if you are feeling a bit queasy still try to eat small, regular meals and plenty of nutritious snacks. I found that starting the day with a banana or plain biscuit, in bed before I got up beat the dreaded morning sickness.

- Although I didn't suffer from morning sickness I did feel a bit queasy in the evenings. With my sense of smell in over-drive I found that if Dave cooked our meals I could stomach it better than having to prepare them myself. Luckily for me on the occasions when I felt rough he was more than happy to do this.

- I also discovered a great company on-line called 'MumsTheWord' and amongst other things I bought some sweets called 'Preggie pop drops' that helped with sickness as well.

Sleep deprivation...

Wednesday 12th December

Dave and I had an appointment with the Citizens Advice Bureau as we were still waiting for our managing agents to fix our ceiling - I was trying so hard not to let all of this get on top of me but it was difficult. As we sat in the office the smell of gloss paint wafted in and I realised they were painting the hallway. I moved my chair so that I was practically sitting on the window sill and tried not to stress about paint fumes. Cheryl my Reiki practitioner had me down to a 'T' when she said I worry about worrying. It was as if no sooner had I solved one source of stress and yet another hopped into its place.

When we got back to the flat we were shocked to see builders up on the roof. When we asked if they were fixing it the guy said, 'Not really luv, just plugging holes!' which didn't instil a huge amount of confidence!

Saturday 15th December

The last couple of nights our neighbour above had kept us awake with the noise from her TV set. At 5 am this morning she had The Spice Girls blaring on one of the music channels which she didn't turn off despite us banging a broom on the ceiling and then her door. I eventually fell asleep but woke a short time later feeling sleep deprived and emotional. I didn't feel pregnant anymore; even my boobs seemed back to normal which was pretty upsetting.

We spent the day tidying the flat as we'd decided that we simply had to get some sleep, so later on we were going to move into our Dover property. My dad called and I ended up crying on the phone to him. He was absolutely lovely, so caring and supportive, which set me off blubbing again.

We moved into the house in Dover and I christened the bath which was sparkling brand new and a luxury after our manky pink suite in Folkestone. Dave had done such an amazing job on the place; it was totally unrecognisable from the 1960's time warp it had been stuck in. Everything felt so new and clean, not to mention quiet. We snuggled down for the night only to discover our mattress had a puncture. How I longed for a real bed! Dave taped it up; we turned the lights off and hoped for the best.

Sunday 16th December

Wow, last night was the best night's sleep I'd had in ages - and the bed even managed to stay semi-inflated.

We went to Tesco and bought lots of healthy food as well as a new mattress - this was our 3rd since the flood!

We spent the rest of the day sorting out the kitchen and cleaning the cupboards - as although they were new they had sawdust, drill bits and all manner of instructional leaflets in them. Later on we ate a healthy salad and reflected on how pleased we were that we had moved here at last. Although to anyone looking in - easily done as we had no curtains - it all looked pretty basic with no furniture or even a TV. We just had two camping chairs, a rickety little table and us - blissfully happy to be together in our peaceful, warm, tidy new home.

Tips & things to do

- You may well be feeling an emotional wreck this week, I know I was! Remember it's not the true you but all those pregnancy hormones - PMT magnified a zillion times. Once you realise it is normal to feel this way you won't be so hard on yourself.

- There are lots of great alternative therapies out there that are suitable for during pregnancy - Reflexology, Homeopathy, Acupuncture and Massage to name but a few. Book a session for your favourite one.

- You could treat yourself to a facial, I found my skin was quite spotty around this time - blame those hormones again!

- Your baby's organs start to form as have its tiny fingers, toes and hair follicles.

I feel like I've had a boob job!

Wednesday 19th December

I went to Canterbury today for another Reiki treatment that went really well. Cheryl always seems to say just the right things to me, she commented on how well I looked especially my skin and hair which made me feel great as I had only just been thinking that my hair was in desperate need of a good hairdresser. After my treatment Dave and I popped into town to finish our Christmas shopping off and had a lovely meal together.

Friday 21st December

Dave and I walked along the riverbank to Dover town centre today. We sorted some banking out and then bought veggie burgers for lunch as I had a bit of a craving for them. We also got lots of healthy stuff in and I made a lentil stew for dinner I probably ate too much though as I had such a bad stomach ache afterwards...ouch!

Sunday 23rd December

We had a bit of a busy day yesterday sorting out the house ready for a letting agent to come and view it. She was pretty impressed and seemed to think it would let easily enough. We were also going to get it valued to sell before deciding what to do.

I felt quite rough all day today and my poor boobs were aching as if I'd had a boob job, but on a positive note it was a good sign that I was still pregnant.

Later while Dave finished up some tiling in the kitchen I lay on the mattress in our bedroom, knitting and eating an apple and 'Whizzers' (vegan 'Smarties', in case you wondered).

Monday 24th December

An estate agent came round to value the house today and although he thought it looked amazing and to quote him 'showroom quality' the market had taken a down-turn so we decided to rent it out until things picked up.

We drove to Somerset, to my dad's where we were spending Christmas together. He was pleased to see us and after dinner we stayed up late chatting and watching TV.

Tips & things to do

- Make sure you are happy with your work environment and that you are taking regular breaks etc. If there is anything you are concerned about you could ask your company to do a risk assessment for you.

- Your boobs may feel like they don't belong to you anymore - mine felt as though I had borrowed them from Dolly Parton! Ditch any under-wired bras as they are not suitable to wear during pregnancy and plan a day out to buy some new comfy ones.

- It's amazing how quickly your baby is developing - this week facial features start to form.

- One of my pregnancy must-haves was given to me by a friend, a clever little device that makes the seatbelt in your car much more comfortable without compromising on your safety. Until I got it I had taken to holding the seatbelt so it couldn't dig into my poor boobs or tummy.

Indigestion, indigestion, indigestion...

Wednesday 26th December

We had a lovely Christmas Day yesterday with my dad, I ate so much that it was 6 pm before I had any space for dessert. After exchanging gifts we 'vegged' out in front the TV for the rest the day.

Today Dave and I drove to my mum's for another huge lunch and a belated Christmas with her. Mum was in fine form, she managed to drop a pot of pepper into the lemon meringue pie she was making and when she went to the store cupboard to get some drinks we heard a loud crash and she reappeared covered in gloss paint that she had knocked off the shelf above her! Later when her partner Ian came home, he managed to do the exact same thing, so the entire room soon stank of white spirit. We had a great day, although I did end up with a stomach ache - I wasn't sure if it was from overeating, laughing, being pregnant, or a combination of all three!

Monday 31st December

The last few days had been spent with my dad and driving around visiting family. It was quite manic but lots of fun! We also drove to Exeter to stay with our fabulous friends Tray and Paul, where we were plied with yet more great food and wonderful company.

We spent New Year's Eve at my Aunt and Uncles where my horrible stomach ache returned forcing me to sit dessert out. I saw the New Year in curled up in pain on an armchair.

Tips & things to do

- Even though you may feel hungry all the time, try to eat small regular meals and snacks rather than 3 large meals. My eyes have always been larger than my stomach and I spent so much of my pregnancy with indigestion. Heartburn is another of the joys of pregnancy that you might experience.

- Spend some quality time with your partner, friends and family especially if you are feeling fit and well.

- Your baby's major organs have formed and now fingernails start to grow.

- Nobody else may have noticed a difference in your body shape but you will have. I spent ages standing side-on to a mirror looking at my stomach. It looked as though I had polished off a very large dinner and possibly someone else's too!

- Start to look forward to your 12 week scan - which in most circumstances is the first time you will get to see your baby.

Guinea-pig fiasco...

Wednesday 2nd January

We left my dad's today and headed across country to Cambridgeshire to visit Dave's mum, Janet, and her husband, Tony. The Christmas celebrations continued as we gave each other presents and had a good catch up. They were both very pleased about my pregnancy and were keeping everything crossed for us that this time it went well.

Friday 4th January

We were home again after all our travels but also back to the stresses of day to day things such as letter writing to ask our managing agents when they were going to repair the ceiling in our Folkestone flat. I got so wound up writing to them that for a couple of hours afterwards I had horrible pains that set me worrying afresh as to whether our baby was OK.

Saturday 5th January

I woke up today with a pain in my hip, so I felt pretty sorry for myself. Dave cheered me up by putting a slideshow of our wedding photos on the computer.

In the afternoon I had a bit of a surreal conversation with our tenants in London. They wanted to leave as it appeared they had fallen out big time with the next-door neighbours. They gave a crazy and rambling account of their dogs escaping into the adjoining garden and trying to dig into the neighbours' guinea-pig pen. At which point the neighbours looked out of their window, had a fit and ended up calling the police who arrived on the scene while I was on the phone, to look at the dangerous dogs that had been reported. The tenant went to speak to them while I filled Dave in as he had just been hearing snippets of the conversation, 'dogs, guinea-pig and police'. A few minutes passed and the tenant rang back to say that the police had left once they had ascertained that the guinea-pigs were intact and that the dangerous dogs were in fact tiny dachshunds. The upshot of the whole fiasco was that we were going to have to go through the rigmarole of finding new tenants and would be avoiding the neighbours for a while. Why couldn't things be simple?

Tips & things to do

- You may have your first scan around now - I had mine at week 13. It is exciting but also nerve-wracking waiting to see your baby for the first time.

- Discuss with your partner the tests that you want to take. It is best to read up about them first - most hospitals will give you some leaflets explaining everything when you book your scan.

- Try to get your partner to come along with you as seeing the baby will make him feel much more part of your pregnancy and be a support to you - especially if you're anything like me and have a fear of hospitals!

- Make sure you have plenty of change for the car park; also some hospitals make a small charge if you want a copy of your scan to take home.

- By this week your baby is fully formed making the risks of miscarriage significantly lower than previous weeks. Tooth buds and hair start to grow around this time.

- One of my magazines said at week 12 a baby was approximately the size of a pear. For us this name kind of stuck!

Our baby waved at us!

Wednesday 9th January

I was finding it increasingly difficult not to get stressed out at this time. Between the London tenants threatening not to pay all the rent money they owed and the ceiling saga in Folkestone still dragging on, it wasn't easy!

I also depressed myself by doing our accounts which were not looking too healthy and set us a food budget to stick to.

Dave and I drove to Brighton to check the work that had been done to our flat's water damaged ceiling. We were both so keen to move to Brighton as we totally love the place. Financially we couldn't afford to buy a house, but figured that we could move into the flat and test drive the area to see if it truly lived up to our expectations. The plan was that when the property market picked up that we would be able to sell our London and Folkestone properties - if we could manage to hang in there that long!

At the flat in Brighton we checked the ceiling that had recently been plastered but we weren't that pleased with the standard of the job done, so that was yet another thing to sort out. On a positive note, as we lay on our trusty inflatable mattress in the evening, we chatted for ages about all the things we would like to do to improve the flat. It hadn't had any work done on it, with the exception of a lick of paint, since we bought it some 5 years ago.

Sunday 13th January

I had a terrible stomach ache last night shortly after dinner. I'd always been prone to tummy ache if I didn't eat regularly enough, but this was happening a lot more frequently now I was pregnant. I decided I was going to have to start eating smaller meals, more frequently and earlier in the evening.

We were back at Dover again and on a mission to finish some fiddly little jobs off, like grouting the kitchen tiles. I took a break and phoned Cheryl, my Reiki practitioner. She had been doing some absent healing for me and today when I chatted to her, I told her how worried I was about the following week when we had to go to the hospital for my scan. She said it was entirely natural for us to be scared and apprehensive about it and that it was understandable that after our previous experiences I would be protecting myself by thinking the worst. She promised to do some more absent healing for me and when I came off the phone from her I felt heaps better.

Monday 14th January

I felt sick with nerves at the thought of my hospital appointment. As we drove to London I made sure I ate some sandwiches in the car and had even packed some belongings in case I had to stay in overnight - talk about being pessimistic.

As we waited to hear the results of the scan I could hardly bring myself to look at the monitor. The sonographer put the clear gel on my tummy and Dave and I exchanged a look with each other, as on all the other occasions I had to have an internal scan. Unbelievably as we looked up we could see something on the monitor. We both just assumed it was someone else's scan that hadn't been deleted! The sonographer said, 'There's your baby' and as we looked I found myself crying, but for sheer happiness this time. She spent ages going through everything with us explaining where its little backbone was, its tiny heart pumping away and even counted its fingers and toes - which seemed to come to the correct number! Next she showed us the baby's eyes and brain that looked like a butterfly and finally the stomach. She let us listen to its heart beat (a healthy 150 beats per minute) and all the time Dave and I were in a shocked state of silence. I found myself holding my breath when she explained that she would be doing the nuchal scan to test for Down's syndrome. Now that I knew there was a baby in there I was praying that it was healthy. Thankfully everything seemed OK, even taking into account my age and she informed me the risk had gone down from 1 in 123 to 1 in 864. I held my breath again as she tested for another syndrome and that too had gone down from 1 in 226 to 1 in 1416, although of course there are no guarantees. After that she took some measurements, crown to rump was 68.6mm and she confirmed my due date was 23rd July.

I was in total shock; I had been feeling so negative recently and hadn't allowed myself to start making any plans, so this all felt very strange. The sonographer looked at the screen again and informed us that our baby was dancing - which delighted us, as both Dave and I were dancers! It stretched and placed a little hand near its mouth, then just as the machine was about to be switched off the baby waved - now I know that sounds crazy, but both Dave and the sonographer saw it too…unbelievable! We came away with some amazing pictures, one that looks like a little sardine and another where our baby was sucking its thumb. We both felt totally overwhelmed and after I'd had a blood test we texted and rang our family to tell them the fantastic news. What an absolutely brilliant day, we had waited so long for this and both just felt incredibly happy.

Tuesday 15ᵗʰ January

I was still on a bit of a high from yesterday - I knew we had a long way to go but for me reaching 13 weeks and seeing our baby was a dream come true.

I was trying to be strict with our money - or should I say lack of money - and had made a list of meals for the week. They were all really healthy and within the budget I had set us. After stocking up in Tesco's, where we were very restrained and only bought what was on the shopping list we returned home to crash out. I was so tired but when I read in my book all the changes that were happening in my body and how rapidly our baby was developing it was hardly surprising. We had dinner and a quick tidy up of the house. One of the joys of not having all our belongings with us was that we couldn't get in too much of a muddle.

Tips & things to do

- Nothing can truly prepare you for the emotions you will feel at seeing your baby for the first time. For us because we had such a long journey to get to this stage it felt like we had reached a huge milestone. It is incredibly exciting for your partner to see your baby moving around inside you too. Until this point he has just had to put up with your ever increasing list of maladies which suddenly all seem worth it.

- Your baby can open and close its hands and even suck its thumb which we saw on our scan picture.

- If you haven't done so already you may feel like telling close family and friends your news and possibly your workplace, depending on your situation.

- We made copies of our scan photo for our parents who were thrilled to see the first picture of their future grandchild. I even took a photo of the scan picture with my mobile and had it as a screensaver!

My quest for a bra...

Wednesday 16th January

We had fresh fruit smoothies and cereal for breakfast, yummy! I felt quite hormonal today and the situation with our London tenants was getting to me. It was raining on and off all day so we stayed in and sorted through all our property files. We had decided to get the lease on our flat in Brighton valued as we would love to be able to purchase it from the freeholder - if the price was right - so we booked someone to come around next Tuesday to take a look at the property.

Friday 18th January

I wrote a letter to our London tenants explaining that if they left the property earlier than their contract date and no-one else moved in that they were liable for the money - I was sure that would be well received!

We popped to the supermarket as we had run out of juice and I noticed a book that I had wanted to read for ages - Sophie Kinsella's 'Shopaholic and Baby'. I had been putting off buying it until I knew I truly was still pregnant and later as I made a start on it I found myself laughing out loud.

Saturday 19th January

I haven't been able to put my book down since I bought it and today I finished and started on another light-hearted chick-lit book. Dave drilled a hole through the wall so at last we would have a TV aerial. I got all domestic in the kitchen and made some delicious oat and dark chocolate chip cookies that I had a bit of a fancy for. In the evening when we snuggled up together to watch a DVD I felt a few little pains; I hoped our baby was still hanging in there.

Sunday 20th January

We were woken at 3.30 am by the most almighty crash that sounded like the next door neighbours roof falling off! They were having a loft conversion so it could have been possible. My heart was banging ten to the dozen at the shock of being woken so suddenly, we went to have a look but everything seemed OK although it took ages for me to calm down enough to go back to sleep.

In the afternoon we drove to Folkestone to check on the flat and do some laundry there as we didn't have a washing-machine at Dover. While our clothes were spinning I went to Debenhams to get measured for a new bra as mine no longer fitted. I had ditched all my under-wired ones and at the moment was wearing a sports bra, but it was really uncomfortable. I had been a 34D for as long as I could remember but the sales assistant informed me I now needed a 36D or 38C. I tried on 8 bras and not one of them was much of an improvement on what I was currently wearing which was disappointing. I left the shop bra-less (literally) and found myself almost holding my poor aching boobs as we made our way home.

We popped in on our neighbours to check their loft was still intact after the huge bang in the night - unbelievably they hadn't heard a thing, so we all traipsed up to their loft for a quick look and everything seemed fine, very strange!

Tuesday 22nd January

We spent the morning frantically tidying up the house as we had estate agents coming to give us valuations. It was such a beautiful day and we were both keen to be outside in the sun but forced ourselves to stay in until the house was in showroom condition.

The first agent valued it between £165,000 and £172,000 and the second at a very disheartening £160,000 - if we sold at that price we would make a loss. Once the agent had left I felt like crying, partly because the valuation was so low, especially after all the hard work we'd put into it, and partly because I had hunger pains as they had been there so long. My poor stomach ached for about an hour; I hoped I wouldn't spend my entire pregnancy like this.

Tips & things to do

- Treat yourself to some pregnancy books or baby related fiction. 'Shopaholic and Baby' by Sophie Kinsella had me in stitches. Great for a light-hearted read. My other favourites were Jools Oliver's 'Minus Nine to One' and 'My Bump and Me' by Myleene Klass.

- By this week your baby will have developed their external sex organs making it possible to tell if your baby is a girl or boy.

- If your waist-line is expanding, treat yourself to some maternity clothes. I have listed my favourite stores at the end of the book.

- Make time for some gentle exercise such as walking, yoga or swimming.

The bra saga continues...

Wednesday 23rd January

I had been looking forward to today as we planned on going shopping in Canterbury and I was sure I would finally get some decent bras. It turned into a total fiasco however. I tried on 19 bras in Debenhams and not one even vaguely fitted. By the time I got to Marks & Spencer's I was close to tears, especially when the assistant there told me that I had been measured wrongly which would explain why nothing fitted. I ended up in the changing room with a great stack of boxes of bras feeling the urge to throw the lot of them at the wall. It was quite funny really because I wasn't even being fussy about the colour or style I just wanted something comfy and supportive - was that too much to ask? I eventually settled on a 36F that was recommended and wore it straight away, by the time I got home it was already digging in and when I took it off I had red marks - not good!

Thursday 24th January

The bra saga continued today, I took yesterday's purchase back to the small M&S in Dover, where not surprisingly they didn't have any bras even close to my size so I just got a refund.

Later we drove to Mothercare where once again I was measured and made yet another size this time 32F - how a tape measure could vary so much between stores was beyond my comprehension! The assistant then broke the news that they didn't actually have a single bra my size in stock, I felt like screaming in frustration - surely it shouldn't be this difficult. In the end I bought a 36 DD which wasn't a perfect fit but by then I was determined not to leave the store empty handed.

Friday 25th January

We walked into Dover town centre to sort out some paperwork at the estate agents office. It was nearly 3 pm by the time we made our way back along the riverbank home. I suddenly got a horrendous tummy ache that had me doubled-up in pain and I found it hard walking the rest the way. When we got in I had to lie down for ages until the pains eased off; I was quite mad at myself for being so silly and not eating sooner. Once the pains had gone I had a jacket potato as I was hungry, but even that came back to haunt me - instead of hunger pains I spent the next hour with indigestion - give me a break!

Saturday 26th January

The day started so well, the sun was out and we went to the estate agents again to confirm that we wanted to put the property on the market to sell.

After lunch we drove to Folkestone where we were confronted with a horrible selection of post. The first letter was from the lease valuation company in Brighton saying that their previous quote was wrong and instead of £11,000 it should have been £15,500. The second was from the managing agents in Folkestone telling us that there was nothing they were prepared to do to rectify our ceiling and water damage problems and the final letter was from a debt collection company saying we owed them money for an unpaid water bill.

I spent the rest the day alternating between crying and then worrying about crying and the effects it might have on our baby.

Monday 28th January

We forced ourselves to get up early and made a start on tidying up as my mum and her partner Ian were coming to stay. Before they arrived I telephoned the agents in Brighton and gave them a bit of a grilling about the miscalculation they had made to the freehold valuation. It didn't get me very far as the person I spoke to justified the mistake by blaming his colleague!

Later when mum and Ian arrived we went out for a drink and heard all about their holiday. They were excited to see our scan pictures and as I chatted to mum about all the annoying little things that had been going on recently she really put things into perspective. Her opinion was that we concentrated on making the flat in Brighton nice for us and our baby rather than worrying about trying to raise the money to buy the freehold - that frankly was now way beyond our means.

Tuesday 29th January

I found it hard to sleep last night as I had tummy ache, again! We were up early as our estate agent wanted to take some photos of the house for their website; she already had two viewings lined up for Saturday so fingers crossed she would find a buyer soon.

We went for a jolly to Canterbury with mum and Ian and in the evening they treated us to an absolutely delicious meal in our favourite Chinese restaurant in Folkestone - extra, extra tofu!

Tips & things to do

- Your baby has a fine, downy hair called 'lanugo' covering its body to protect its fine skin. This will disappear later on in your pregnancy.

- Your clever little baby has possibly learnt a new trick this week - as well as thumb-sucking he or she can grab the umbilical cord and use it as its first toy.

- Now you are into the 2nd trimester you will hopefully be feeling less sick and start to get that pregnancy bloom that all the books mention. It was quite some weeks before I felt it I must admit!

- One of my pregnancy books said that I may find my sex drive returned round about now. I must confess we were pretty cautious throughout my entire pregnancy after my miscarriages. I figured we had enough sex leading up to my pregnancy to keep us going for a while - not sure Dave agreed with me on that one!
  If you are unsure seek advice from your doctor or midwife as every pregnancy is different.

- You may experience strange, vivid or in my case the occasional erotic dreams. Hey I may not have been actually having sex but my brain was obviously thinking about it! Again all normal pregnancy symptoms.

- On the subject of dreams you could keep a journal of them if they aren't too blue! As well as cravings, mood and energy levels.

- Take photos of your growing bump and maybe start a video diary.

That sinking feeling...

Wednesday 30th January

I had a stomach ache for ages last night most likely after wolfing down too much Chinese food but it was delicious.

We said our goodbyes to mum and Ian as they were going home and we were off to London for a doctor's appointment.

I think I managed to embarrass myself whilst simultaneously entertaining an entire waiting room full of patients when I mistakenly thought that the receptionist wanted me to give her a urine sample in a plastic zippy bag she was holding. How was that supposed to work? I didn't see the plastic container she had concealed in her other hand.

I was seen by a lovely midwife who announced that my urine was nice and clear, which was good to know and in a bottle and not a bag! She found our baby's heartbeat straight away which was very exciting. I could have listened to it beating away all day; I was half tempted to buy a machine so we could listen at home, but I knew I would drive myself nuts with it. I told the midwife about my recurring stomach ache and she suggested I got it checked out at the hospital.

This seemed like a good idea until nearly 3 hours had passed in A&E and I was about to get hunger pains again. The doctor I saw prodded my tummy a bit and said it was most likely gastritis and not to worry about it; she recommended I took Gaviscon if I got it again.

Saturday 2nd February

We spent ages sorting out things at the house in Dover before we could finally leave for Brighton. We went via Folkestone so we could do some laundry there and hang it up; I couldn't wait for the day when we actually had a washing-machine in the house we lived in. We then ended up going back to Dover as Dave had forgotten his trainers and he needed them for his run the next day...growl!

It was 5 pm by the time we got to Brighton and as we were both starving we went straight to Wagamama for dinner. I think it was too late for me as I had only eaten a few mouthfuls when my stomach started aching once more. We went to our flat and Dave unpacked the car while I lay curled up on the floor by the radiator crying. About an hour later the pains had eased off thankfully so we blew up our inflatable mattress and settled down for the night. The pub across the road from us was really noisy so it was hard to get off to sleep despite us both being tired. Just as I was drifting off I felt a sinking sensation and realised our mattress was going down; poor Dave ended up having to blow it up 5 times during the night - with me still laying on it!

Sunday 3rd February

Last night Dave and I had seriously started to doubt our decision to move to Brighton after all the noise keeping us awake, but today everything seemed better. Dave went on a run and I went to the local organic supermarket, Infinity Foods, just a few streets away and bought yoghurt, cereal and French bread for breakfast. I could most definitely get used to being able to walk everywhere, as all our previous homes had been a car-ride away from civilisation, here in Brighton everything we could possibly need was close by. After breakfast we wandered to Laura Ashley and came away with some wallpaper samples to try out in what will hopefully soon be our bedroom. The absolute highlight of the day was that we finally ordered ourselves a bed. It was going to take a while for it to be delivered which would give us chance to decorate the room first. I couldn't wait to sleep on a real bed again!

In the evening we went to our favourite vegetarian restaurant Terre à Terre for dinner and despite stuffing myself silly with their gorgeous food I miraculously didn't get a stomach ache...Yay!

Monday 4th February

We went to Neal's Yard in the morning and I bought some 'slippery elm' which is supposed to help with stomach aches. I knew I was allowed to take Gaviscon but I would prefer to use a more natural product if possible.

From there we walked to a store that specialised in natural, organic, vegan paints that were totally safe for me and our baby. The girl in there was helpful and once we had decided on what wallpaper to use in the bedroom she would mix us up a paint to match. It was such a civilised place to shop, complete with a comfy sofa to relax on whilst browsing through colour charts.

We then went to Argos to take back a replacement mattress we'd bought as that seemed to have a puncture too. Dave fixed our original blow-up bed with a puncture repair kit from a pound shop so hopefully we would sleep better tonight. In the evening I got my usual tummy ache and gave the 'slippery elm' a go; it was pretty disgusting and I'm not sure I mixed it up properly as it was quite lumpy, yuk!

Tuesday 5th February

We were up and out early as I had a 'booking in' appointment at my doctor's in London. I couldn't wait until we actually made the move to Brighton and I could hopefully get a doctors surgery within walking distance instead of the major schlep we had to keep making.

I was disappointed when we finally got to London and found that my appointment wasn't the 'booking in' I'd been expecting, as the receptionist had made a mistake. The doctor did however let us listen to our baby's heartbeat and told me the blood and urine tests I had done previously were both fine.

Before driving back to Dover we popped in on our lovely friends Emma and Al who recently had a baby boy. He is called Connor and is absolutely gorgeous, I had a cuddle of him then Emma handed him to Dave, who at first looked a little shell-shocked as he had never held a baby before but he turned out to be a total natural...phew!

Tips & things to do

- Your baby is developing so quickly, by now he or she can swallow, hiccup and kick - although you most likely won't feel any movements yet.

- Every time you go to see your doctor or midwife they will test a urine sample to check for protein, sugar or bacteria in it. I worried every time I took the test, but felt hugely reassured afterwards when told everything was fine.

- You may want to buy some lotions and potions to help prevent stretch marks. I think whether you get them or not is largely down to luck and genes but you may as well slather yourself in something luxurious. I swore by the 'Mama Mio' range and started using the 'Tummy Rub Stretch Mark Oil' - not cheap, but worth every penny. I alternated it with 'Sanctuary Mum to Be Collagen Boosting Body Butter' - mmmh gorgeous! The Sanctuary also has lovely bath salts in their Mum-to-be range that smell devine.

- Your skin may change slightly; if you have moles or freckles they might change colour or shape a bit. If you're worried speak to your doctor about it.

- Another lovely pregnancy symptom you could get around about now is the appearance of spider veins on your face and legs. In most cases they fade after your baby is born.

Vegan paint dilemma...

Wednesday 6th February

We were woken by the phone just before 9 am; it was Chris the builder who was going to fix the ceiling of our Folkestone flat at last. We arranged to meet him at the flat to show him what needed doing - although in my opinion it was fairly obvious!

We packed some more bits and pieces in the car to take back to Dover and eventually on to Brighton. In the afternoon I wrote a couple of letters to the managing agents and Valuation Company in Brighton - It was all very time consuming. I felt a bit hormonal today - it was annoying that we knew where we wanted to be but obstacles kept preventing us from getting there. Dave and I just wanted to get to Brighton and make a start on getting the flat ready for us and our baby.

Friday 8th February

We drove to Brighton last night and today went on a quest for a new kitchen for the flat, as the one in there was decidedly scummy. All the cupboard doors were hanging off and the cooker was an ancient stand alone electric model circa 1980. The only thing holding it together was probably the quantity of grease and burnt food stuck to it; I long for the day we meet tenants with a cleaning fetish!

We were going to walk to Howdens Joinery but fortunately decided to catch a train as it turned out to be miles away. We had a browse at their sample kitchen cupboards and were delighted to see that they had brought out a new range which was reasonably priced but also very contemporary. We booked an appointment for a designer to come over on Monday to measure up and give us a quote.

After lunch we returned to the eco paint store where it took ages for the paint to get mixed to the same shade as the background colour on the Laura Ashley wallpaper. As soon as we got in Dave cracked on with painting the ceiling, while I went for a wander around the shops.

Sunday 10th February

I woke at 6.15 am to hear the front door closing as Dave left for a run - mad man!

I stayed in bed snoozing; I didn't have any stomach ache last night and felt great today. Dave returned at 8.30 am and we had breakfast together.

Afterwards he made a start on what would be our bedroom and told me to make the most of the sunshine by taking a walk. I didn't want to stand in the way of a man on a D.I.Y. mission so I skedaddled and found a sunny spot on the beach. As I sat there I felt such a wave of happiness wash over me, something I hadn't experienced in a while, what with all the constant property dilemmas we'd had recently. I started re-reading Jools Oliver's pregnancy book and allowed myself to get a bit excited about our little baby and our new life we would shortly be starting here in beautiful Brighton by the sea.

Monday 11th February

Oh my goodness, what a shock I had this morning when I crept downstairs while Dave was sleeping to view his handy-work in the bedroom. The paint hadn't dried yet, despite all the windows being left open overnight and worse still, what had dried looked terrible. On the window sills our lovely organic, vegan paint had some kind of a reaction to what was on there previously and the result was a thick greenish skin not unlike the one that used to turn my stomach on the school dinners custard we were expected to eat. Dave had spent ages putting masking tape around the glass on the windows to prevent paint from getting on them, but the paint had run so badly it looked as if someone had thrown a bucket of milk at them.

We decided to return to the paint shop to ask them their advice - the guy was great and he actually came back with us to see for himself. He said in 15 years he had never seen anything like it and offered to replace the paint as he thought it was faulty, he even threw in a free paint scraper and some undercoat for good measure. Poor Dave was not a happy bunny as it was going to be a nightmare getting the gooey mess of paint off, then he would have to start the whole process again. We were both regretting the decision we made in the first place of not using undercoat to save time and money - that had proven to be a false economy!

We found a doctors surgery less than 5 minutes walk from our flat and made an appointment with the nurse to register there. She took both of our blood pressures, heights and weights and we left feeling pleased to have found a surgery that didn't involve us having to take in the delights of the M25.

The Howdens' designer came over in the afternoon, measured our kitchen and made some suggestions for the best use of the space we had.

Dave managed to fill the car with all the old carpet from the bedroom (I was extremely glad to say goodbye to that) but we had run out of time to take it to the tip. I was absolutely exhausted from our busy day and crashed out. Dave stayed up as an old friend of ours was coming over to stay the night. Dames didn't arrive till 11 pm and he slept on our spare inflatable mattress in the disaster zone we called our bedroom. Before I fell asleep I told Dave to warn Dames not to sleep too close to the wall in case his hair got stuck to the wet paint on the skirting boards!

Tuesday 12th February

I caught up with Dames in the morning, he had made it through the night without getting stuck to any of our paintwork and thought the whole thing was hilarious. I whizzed off to a doctor's appointment while the boys went to a flat Dames owns nearby to do some work on it - I made sure they didn't take any vegan paint with them!

Once again the appointment I had wasn't the elusive 'booking in' appointment I was expecting - at this rate I might have given birth before I got booked in! But on the plus side I got to listen to my baby's heartbeat again.

I was told that I needed to make an appointment with a midwife who was based in a children's clinic nearby. That suited me no end as I was not keen sitting in the waiting room with lots of poorly people coughing and sneezing everywhere - there's my Dot Cotton-like hypochondria rearing its ugly little head again. The children's clinic was lovely and I managed to make an appointment for next Wednesday.

I popped into the Jog Shop to buy Dave some running socks and a magazine for Valentine's Day.

I went in a lovely baby shop near our flat called 'JoJo Maman Bébé' it is an oasis of all things baby. I tried on a few bras in their changing room and entertained myself immensely with a delightful little tie-on bump that was hanging in there. I found myself twirling in front the mirror with the bump under my top - strange to think I would have one for real soon! I treated myself to a bra that felt pretty comfy...Yay!

For dinner we went out with Dames to a fabulous vegan pub nearby called The George where we had a great meal and a catch-up. I had the most amazing vegetable fajitas with all the trimmings and luckily managed not to get tummy ache.

Tips & things to do

- If you have any painting or D.I.Y. that needs doing on your property try to use a low or no-voc paint and keep the rooms well ventilated. Better still get your partner or a professional to do it while you find somewhere nice to relax and put your feet up.

- This week your baby starts to develop some fat and the lungs continue forming.

- You may feel some pangs as your ligaments in your tummy stretch to accommodate your ever increasing uterus.

- The area around your nipples called the areola might darken in colour and get larger as your boobs just keep on growing!

- I did panic this week when I read somewhere that you could expect to get something called a 'linea nigra', which is a dark line down your abdomen or a 'mask of pregnancy' on your face, that is a darkening of the skin and looks a bit like a butterfly in shape. Thankfully I didn't get either but even if you do they will fade once your baby is born ... phew!

- Try - if you can - to train yourself to sleep on your left side as it is better for your blood supply to your baby. I found it quite comfy wedging a pillow between my knees and also behind my back to stop me rolling into my usual pre-pregnancy sleep position.

Those pesky hormones again...

Wednesday 13th February

We walked to Dames' flat in the morning and I sat out in the back garden while the boys beavered away, fixing the back door and the bathroom.

I left them to it and wandered back to the North Laine, stopping at Infinity Cafe where I picked up the most delicious salad to eat on the beach. I think my eyes were bigger than my stomach however, as shortly after I had demolished a big slice of tofu chocolate cheesecake I started to get a tummy ache. I went back to the flat and thankfully the pains subsided in about half an hour. I really needed to get a handle on maybe eating little and often if I wanted to get through my pregnancy without too much indigestion.

The boys came back and Dames said goodbye as he had a train to catch home. Dave and I ate at the pub again as we both felt too tired to cook and neither of us were brave enough anyway to eat anything apart from baked beans off our decrepit cooker.

Thursday 14th February

I woke up and experienced an unpleasant shooting pain inside when I went to the toilet I hoped our baby was OK.

Luckily it passed; I made a mental note to mention it to the midwife.

As it was Valentine's Day I gave Dave his card and pressies which he really liked. He felt bad because in all the madness of trying to leave Dover he accidently left my card and gift there - something to look forward to anyway. We ate in the pub again; I couldn't wait until we got our new kitchen as although it was great eating out, at this rate it would cost us a fortune.

Friday 15th February

Oh dear, my hormones definitely got the better of me. Dave and I went for a drive to Wickes to scope out some laminate flooring for the flat but we didn't see anything we particularly liked. On the way back we stopped at a cafe for lunch. It was a typical greasy spoon that served breakfast all day. I ended up feeling quite tearful however, when the waitress couldn't/wouldn't tell me whether the veggie sausages were vegan or not. I didn't think my request was unreasonable as all she needed to do was nip in the kitchen and read the packet. So as Dave tucked into an enormous plate of sausages, eggs, beans, mushrooms and toast I sat moodily pushing my baked beans and dry toast around the plate with tears threatening to spring out my eyes at any given moment. Feeling like a petulant little child I remained sulking until Dave suggested he dropped me at Infinity Cafe to pick up a take-out salad. I knew I was being silly getting upset over something as petty as a sausage but I just couldn't stop myself...pesky hormones!

The day improved no end when later, after my scrummy dose of healthy salad I went for my first hairdresser's appointment in ages. I had read on the internet that it was fine to highlight your hair during pregnancy but where I had experienced 2 miscarriages I hadn't wanted to take the chance and had left it for ages; hence my hair was looking pretty sorry for itself.

Three hours later I felt like a new woman thanks to the expertise of Marc my hairdresser - it's amazing what a bit of a snip, blow-dry and colour can do for a girl's self-esteem.

Sunday 17th February

Dave was up and out early to do the Brighton half-marathon. I walked to Madeira Drive to watch the runners start then made my way towards The Pavilion to see them. They were all so quick that I missed them there and at every part of the race, I seemed to get there just after they had all run past! I did eventually make it back down to the seafront in time to catch Dave pass through the finish line in a good time of 2 hours and 6 minutes.

After a cold bath - for Dave - and a late breakfast/ early lunch for us both we made our way to The Pavilion as I had some free tickets for a Wedding Fayre they were hosting. It was hard to believe almost two years had past since we were married there and it was so lovely being back. This time we did the full guided tour and also had a wander around the Wedding Fayre that was set up in The Red Drawing Room, where we held our blessing and also the beautiful William IV Room, where are reception had been...how sentimental are we!

Monday 18th February

While Dave glossed the bedroom (again) I went to Infinity Foods supermarket and bought freshly baked bread and vegan bacon. We had started cooking at the flat on our camping stove, which was a bit of a military operation if you wanted more than one thing cooked at a time, but great for fry-ups.

I busied myself for hours in the afternoon going through a suitcase of my old clothes, picking out what I could still wear and what needed to go up in the loft. I ended up giving Dave a bit of a mini fashion show - much to his amusement. I found myself getting excited when things didn't fit, as up until recently I hadn't really felt as though my body looked much different than usual, maybe just a bit less toned. But as I struggled to do yet another popper up on my favourite combat trousers the realisation started to sink in that I was actually pregnant and not just flabby!

I got excited again in the evening when I was chatting on the phone to Emma and she said that she was starting to put baby clothes aside for us. I felt so happy, it's been a long, hard journey and at times we thought we would never reach this point. I was keeping everything crossed that this time it was a case of '3rd time's the charm!'

Tuesday 19th February

Dave went on a run while I sorted through some boxes marked 'kitchen stuff', although our kitchen was non-existent. We went to Screwfix, Dave's favourite place and kind of an Argos for builders. After searching through the magazine we found some laminate flooring at a good price and ordered some to be delivered in a few days time.

I felt so happy, at last everything was falling into place and better still I got through the day with no tummy ache. Later when I lay down I noticed that my stomach was looking huge for me and I wondered how much bigger it would get?

Tips & things to do

- You may well be feeling hormonal and have days when even the tiniest of things, sausages even, send you scuttling for the box of tissues.

- Although your baby's ears are not fully formed he or she may still respond to sound so talk or sing to them. I had a little repertoire of songs I sang in the bath to Pear ranging from 'I love you baby I do' sung to the tune of 'We love you England we do' to 'Kick me baby, baby, kick me' and that old favourite from 'Grease' that I slightly changed the words to, 'You're the one that I want, you are the one I want, ooh, ooh, ooh baby!' Dave joked that at around this time our baby probably learnt how to put its fingers in its ears!

- Your uterus is about the size of a melon - I'm hoping Honeydew or Cantaloupe and not Watermelon!

- You may feel light-headed and a bit forgetful. It's great to have a proper excuse at last! I found writing things down helped.

- You could look at booking a holiday or mini-break for you and your partner.

Strange pains...

Wednesday 20th February

We went to the children's clinic to see the midwife today and were disappointed when we discovered it still wasn't the ever elusive 'booking in' appointment. Apparently they needed an hour time slot for that and I'd only been allocated half an hour. The midwife was lovely and sensing our frustration made a start on the 'booking in' paperwork anyway. To our delight she found our baby's heartbeat straight away and said it was nice and strong... that was just always my favourite part of the appointment.

We popped out to get some more paint and went to the supermarket. At around 4 pm I started to feel some pains not unlike period pains that lasted until 11 pm. I got a bit upset as I wasn't sure if that was normal or not and my left hip went into a stitch, as if I had trapped something, about 4 times during the evening. Dave was such a star; he rubbed my hip and legs and pampered me all night.

Thursday 21st February

I had a good nights sleep and woke at 8.30 am feeling a bit better. I tried ringing the children's clinic to ask about my pains but just got their answer phone so I felt a bit stressed out; although the pains were not as bad as last night they were still there.

In the afternoon I went for a walk while Dave painted the hallway. As I reached the supermarket I was approached by a couple of girls with a cameraman who asked if they could interview me for a TV programme they were making about women's health. I agreed, thinking that with everything I have gone through recently that I would be able to come up with a few gems of wisdom regarding pregnancy and miscarriages. They started rolling the camera and the girl doing the interview asked me, 'So have you ever heard of female ejaculation?' Well, you could have knocked me down with a feather I didn't see that one coming! The street suddenly seemed full of people all waiting in silence to hear my answer. I must have gone scarlet with embarrassment and mumbled that, yes, I had heard of it. The rest of the questions were even more cringe worthy ranging from, 'Have you had it happen to you?' to 'Would you discuss it with a friend?' That would be a no and a no! I was so glad when they finally turned the camera off and I could make my escape.

Friday 22nd February

I was woken by the phone ringing at 8.30 am; it was a midwife returning my call from yesterday. She said I should take a sample of urine to the doctor's to check I didn't have an infection - apparently it could cause premature labour in some women. My wee was so dark in colour I had myself convinced that something was wrong. I got quite tearful in the doctor's room as I waited to find out. The doctor was lovely and said everything was absolutely fine and took time to explain where our baby was and answered all our questions.

In the evening we left Brighton and made our way back to Dover via the flat in Folkestone. I chickened out of going inside to check the state of the ceiling as I just didn't need the stress. Dave went in while I waited tensely in the car, when he returned he said that although it wasn't finished it looked a whole lot better...phew!

Saturday 23rd February

I slept well last night; Dover was so quiet in comparison to Brighton, but saying that I couldn't wait to move there properly. We drove to the flat in Folkestone to do some laundry and dropped the keys at the letting agents, as the ceiling was nearly fixed we could look at letting it - finally! The car had been playing up recently so Dave bought a battery charger, which would hopefully do the trick. We packed a lot into the day; I spoke to my mum on the phone and we sorted out some letters and paperwork on the computer before crashing out for the night.

Sunday 24th February

A while back Dave bought another Volvo on ebay which was just as well because the one we'd been driving had finally given up the ghost. Today we were due to sell it for spare parts to some guy. Dave drove over to Folkestone to try to charge the battery but the metal arm on the bonnet had snapped so he couldn't open it. Then the guy who was going to buy it from us rang to say his van had broken down en-route so he couldn't make it anyway!

While Dave was having fun and games with the car I packed more of our belongings up to take to Brighton and dried our laundry on the radiators at Dover. I felt so good today, lots of energy and no pains for a change. We had a lovely roast for dinner and Dave packed the new Volvo - well, it's pretty old, but new to us! We didn't get to Brighton until 11.15 pm, I was so glad to snuggle up in bed until the dreaded tummy ache struck again. I tossed and turned in pain until 2 am when I finally succumbed to taking some Gaviscon which seemed to do the trick.

Tuesday 26th February

I was exhausted still from our busy weekend so just took things easy. I went to Infinity Foods and bought some freshly baked sundried tomato bread to have with our veggie bacon for lunch. As I walked back I felt some more strange pulling pains - I had thought the 2nd trimester was supposed to be the easy one. It was hard to carry on as normal when my body was doing all manner of weird things to me.

I spent the rest of the day making phone calls as we were connected at last and cooked a tasty lentil stew for dinner - no tummy ache, yippee!

Tips & things to do

- You are practically at the half-way point now of your pregnancy, well done!

- Your baby starts to get more active about now, so you may feel him or her moving around. It feels a bit like you have butterflies in your tummy and is called 'quickening'.

- You may have an anomaly scan around this time to check how your baby is developing. Some hospitals will tell you the sex of your baby if you want to know. Have a chat with your partner as to whether you would like to be told, or if you want to wait and have a surprise.

- All my books and magazines stressed the importance of doing pelvic floor exercises - especially if after the birth you want to be in full control of your bladder when you cough or sneeze! To do them you squeeze the same muscles you would to stop yourself having a wee. I made myself do a few every time I washed my hands.

- There are lots of things that are stopping you from getting a good night's sleep - indigestion and heartburn being the top two culprits. I also found that when I finally did drift off, I frequently woke myself up by snoring - either that or Dave was digging me in the ribs to shut me up!

- One of my magazines referred to the baby as a 'tiny tenant', this cracked Dave and me up. We were seriously hoping that our 'tiny tenant' wouldn't be as much trouble to us as our adult tenants seemed to be!

The week we finally moved to Brighton & got a proper bed...

Wednesday 27th February

I actually slept really well last night for a change. While Dave went on a run I did the washing-up and sorted out our laundry. We were going to have to use a laundrette for a while until we got our own washing-machine.

I went to get my mum a mother's day card in WHSmith and ended up in a huge queue behind 30 people - I counted! I got so hot and flustered and was glad when I finally made it to the front.

When I got back to the flat Dave had made a start on laying some laminate flooring in the hallway. I gave him a hand, mostly in a supervisory role, it looked great and a major improvement on the manky old carpet. We got halfway down the hallway when Dave discovered that the front door step was totally rotten. That threw a bit of a spanner in the works as it needed replacing before we carried on with the rest of the flooring. I was up for doing a bit of a bodge job and ignoring it but Dave pointed out that if he finished the floor before fixing the step he would end up damaging the laminate when he sawed the old door step out...Oh how frustrating!

Thursday 28th February

Dave and I got stuck into laying the floor in the bedroom today; we were leaving the hallway until Dave had bought some wood to fix the door step. I helped by laying out the pieces ready for Dave to cut and then by holding the end so we could click each section together. It was incredibly satisfying seeing each strip completed, I couldn't wait to see it totally finished.

At 3.30 pm I had another midwife's appointment and handed in all my completed paperwork so I was booked in, at last. She took some blood, which was fine as I didn't look, and told me I would need to pick up the results from my doctors surgery next week. We got to hear our baby's heartbeat, I always felt so reassured hearing its little heart galloping away ten to the dozen, it made it all seem more real.

Friday 29th February

Dave finished the floor in our bedroom and it looked amazing. I did my usual routine of Infinity Foods Cafe for a take-out salad - I was hooked on the tahini dressing they put on it, it had such a moreish taste I could have drunk it. I suppose there could be worse things to be craving at least it wasn't raw steak or coal!

I bought some beautiful wallpaper from Laura Ashley called 'Pavilion' that was remarkably similar to the hand-painted wallpaper adorning the rooms at The Royal Pavilion where Dave and I were married. It was quite expensive so we planned to just paper the chimney breast in the bedroom. My mum, who is a great wallpaperer, had offered to do it for us, as Dave and I had never hung paper with a pattern in it before - wood chip was more our speciality!

The highlight of the day was the delivery of our bed. We assembled it and found it filled practically the entire bedroom. We were so looking forward to sleeping on it.

We braved the rain to take a trip up the high street to buy some blinds for the bedroom windows - as the world and his wife could see in. Our flat had a strange little upside down arrangement, with the bedroom and bathroom on the ground floor and the living room and kitchen upstairs. Below the bedroom we had a tiny little studio flat we let out to tenants.

Dave spent ages fixing the blinds as each slat needed trimming on both ends, a time consuming job to say the least. I got my tummy ache again, this time I took some Gaviscon straight away and was nearly sick...not good!

Saturday 1st March

It was really late, or should I say early morning, before I finally got off to sleep. It seemed even noisier outside than usual, which may have been because we were now at street level, so even closer to the pub opposite. In the end Dave went to his tool box and we both equipped ourselves with industrial ear muffs - how hilarious we must have looked! On a positive note our new bed was fantastic! It felt strange being so high up after the endless months of being on the floor on our inflatable mattress. The bed had come at just the right time as I was beginning to find it quite hard to get my ever-increasing-in-size-body up in the morning and the last couple of weeks I had been rolling off the mattress and then slowly getting up from a crawling position.

We spent a while filling the car with rubbish to take to the tip before driving to Folkestone. It was 7.30 pm by the time we got there and I slept in the car while Dave nipped in to put some laundry in the machine to pick up tomorrow.

We drove to Dover via Tesco's for some groceries for dinner and by 10 pm I was bathed and in bed - blinking inflatable mattress again!

Sunday 2nd March

We returned to Folkestone to see off Tony (our car named after my dad who always drives a Volvo). We both were quite sad to see him go - albeit he didn't actually drive away as he was totally broken down. He was loaded onto a trailer, while Dave and I reminisced about all the fun places we had visited in him. I was about to cry when Dave pointed out that he would most likely get used as spare parts or as I put it get rein-CAR-nated!

After waving goodbye to the car - I know we are nuts! Dave went on a run while I vacuumed the flat ready for tenants to view it. I did loads of laundry, making the most of having a machine at hand and soon was exhausted and famished. I went up the high street in search of something I could cook that wouldn't involve any cooking utensils as we didn't have any at the flat. All I came up with was rather uninspiring hash browns and barbeque sauce that I suddenly had a craving for. I had eaten 9 of them by the time Dave returned and saved me from stuffing the rest of the packet.

Monday 3rd March

We spent all day packing the dribs and drabs we still had strewn around the place to take with us to Brighton. We would have moved 4 times in less than a year, and although we were being quite ruthless with throwing away stuff we didn't need, the reality was that we were moving from a 3 bedroom house with a loft and garage to a 1 bedroom flat with a tiny loft and no garage to stash things in. I thought our Brighton pad might well burst at the seams.

We also found time to pop into town to give the estate agents a bit of a kick up the bottom about the lack of viewings they'd had for our property so far. The market had taken a bit of a downturn so we might well return to plan A which was to let it.

My mum drove from Somerset to help us with the move and arrived at 4.30 pm so we had a cuppa and a catch up. Then while I prepared dinner Dave and mum filled the cars with our junk, I mean belongings!

Tuesday 4th March

What a demanding day; it took ages to finish packing our Volvo convoy and despite my placing everything in order in the hallway so we would know where everything was mum and Dave just chucked it all in the cars willy-nilly. I left most of the hard graft of lifting and carrying to them while I tidied and cooked; after all an army marches on its stomach, well Dave's certainly does!

I went with mum in her car so we could chat on route and we got to Brighton just before 3 pm. I guarded the cars while Dave and mum lugged all the things into our flat; I couldn't believe that we had finally moved here officially. Mum loved the flat - bless her for being able to see beyond the mountains of boxes and dodgy decor. It took some major jiggling around to clear enough floor space in the living room to blow the bed up for her to sleep on - mercifully we didn't hear any huge crashes in the night of anything toppling on top of her!

Tips & things to do

- You may start feeling a bit breathless as everything moves up and outwards in your body. Take it easy and if possible let others take charge.

- Your uterus has moved all the way to your navel making you want to wee even more frequently - I bet you're thinking, is that actually possible! I trained myself to go to the toilet in the night with my eyes half shut so I wouldn't wake fully.

- Your tummy button may have gone from an 'innie' to an 'outie'. I found this particularly fascinating!

- Your baby's senses are developing and he or she will start to gain a protective coating over its skin called 'vernix'.

WEEK 21

We find out the sex of our baby...

Wednesday 5th March

Mum and I spent most the day wallpapering the wall in our bedroom. I thought I was being terribly helpful and clever by cutting several pieces the correct length ready for her to stick up. That was until we realised that we needed to match the pattern up and I had succeeded in chopping the head off the bird at the top - a bit of an expensive mistake at nearly £50 a roll! Once we had sussed it out we got on really well and the finished wall looked magnificent. I just couldn't stop admiring it, it was like having a favourite piece of artwork on display and as I fiddled with the dimmer switch it even looked great in subdued lighting, with the background taking on a slightly pearl-like glow...Lovely!

Thursday 6th March

We were all up early today; mum as she needed to get back for work and us to go to the hospital for a scan.

It was extremely stressful trying to park at the hospital; we ended up with just 7 minutes till my allocated appointment time and still no joy. Dave dropped me off while he continued playing musical car spaces with everyone else in Brighton. As I sat in the waiting room I started to worry that Dave would miss the appointment and was considering asking to swap slots with someone else. This would have been a good plan but for the fact I was the only person waiting! On the walls there were several photocopies of the same letter informing parents-to-be that if they wished to know the sex of their baby to ask at the very beginning of the appointment. I was called through and Dave came running in shortly after. The sonographer got to work making all the checks and taking measurements of our baby to confirm it was developing well, while Dave and I held our breath hoping for the best. She announced everything seemed to be normal which was a huge relief and then asked if we would like to know the sex of our baby. Dave and I hadn't had a chance to discuss whether we did or not, what with all the madness of moving and then my mum staying over. I said to the sonographer that we would only want to know if she was really certain. Without saying how sure or not she was she suddenly zoomed in on the scan and exclaimed, 'There's his penis!' Dave and I looked at the scan and then at each other in total shock; somehow being told we were having a boy made it all so much more real. Up till this point I was half expecting to be told, 'You're having a kitten or a monkey!' The sonographer printed off some of the scan photos but disappointingly they were not as clear as the 12 week ones - I guess there was less room in there for Pear to pose!

The rest of the day I remained in shock and felt quite emotional. I was so excited to be having a boy, especially as when I was little I used to beg my mum to make me an older brother and when she said it wasn't possible

I thought she was being mean! Somehow though I thought Dave and I were both expecting our baby to be a girl, for silly reasons really, I'm quite a girly girl and also I used to teach little girls so felt more confident around them, boys were a bit of an unknown territory for me. As the realisation started to sink in that were actually having a baby I also began worrying that I wouldn't be a good enough mum.

Friday 7th March
I was still feeling a bit emotional today. I showed Dave a dress I had been planning on buying to wear for his mum's 70th birthday celebration next week but it didn't look as nice today as the last time I tried it on. In the end I found a skirt and top in our wardrobe that had been packed away for so long I forgot I had it - It had a bold red and white pattern, with a gypsy style top and skirt with an elasticated waistband - so it was a comfortable fit - and a lovely handkerchief hemline. As I posed in front of the wardrobe mirror, checking every angle, I was pleased to see it really showed off my gorgeous baby bump. I felt so happy that I was pregnant and couldn't wait to show Pear off to our family at the meal.

Saturday 8th March
Dave went to buy some wood to fix our rotten front door step. He had fun and games trying to fit the new piece in as it wasn't exactly the same size. He thought I had lost the plot totally when I assured him it would be fine once he had put some sellotape on it! My pregnancy brain had really kicked in, I knew that I wanted to say cement and yet sellotape just popped out.

Sunday 9th March

Dave went out on a long run - 18 miles - as he was doing The London Marathon soon, while I did some secret shopping for his birthday. He already had part of his present from me; some new trainers as his old ones were literally falling apart at the seams. I bought him some trainer socks, sports gels and 'pain au chocolate' for his birthday breakfast as well as a small chocolate birthday cake, he would be needing another long run after all that!

I called my mum in the evening and told her our news on finding out that Pear was a boy. She said she had guessed by the shape I was - apparently if you're carrying a boy it shows more round the back whereas a girl shows more at the front. I joked with her that I was offended she was implying my bum was big!

Monday 10th March

It was Dave's birthday and I made sure he was duly pampered with breakfast and pressies in bed. There was severe winds and rain all day so we stayed indoors for most of it. When we did venture out in the afternoon I felt a bit rough. I didn't want to spoil Dave's birthday treat, I had booked a meal at 'Food for Friends' in the evening, so I had a lie down and a nap for an hour and felt so much better. The restaurant had decorated our table with birthday confetti which was a nice touch. Our food was delicious, I had a vegetable stir-fry on a seaweed base and Dave opted for a tasty vegetable curry. For dessert I had a selection of vegan ice cream in a handmade brandy basket and Dave had a coffee... yummy!

Tuesday 11th March

We had a bit of a nightmare day today. The tenants in London (remember the guinea-pig fiasco) were refusing to pay their last month's rent and the company that did the inventory check-out had sent us a ridiculously basic letter, so we were none the wiser as to what sort of a state they had left the place in. I spent/wasted pretty much the entire day on the phone. I spoke to a particularly snooty woman from the inventory company who patronised me so much that I ended up in tears and Dave had to take over.

Tips & things to do

- You may start feeling clumsy as your tummy grows throwing your weight off balance especially if you favour high heels.

- When deciding if you want to know the sex of your baby it sometimes helps to list the pros and cons. Our pros were that by knowing we could prepare ourselves better, we could start talking to our baby as a he or she rather than 'it' and we also felt that by knowing we would bond sooner with our baby. The only con we had was if the hospital wasn't certain as it would be a shock to be told the wrong sex - especially if we had been out shopping for blue or pink baby wear.

- Your baby is continuing to gain weight and can swallow the amniotic fluid he or she is surrounded by - this will help the development of the digestive system.

We feel Pear wiggle!

Wednesday 12th march

It took ages to get off to sleep last night as I had stomach ache, it wasn't as bad as usual but enough to keep me awake.

Dave went on a run and when he got back in we received a phone call from our London tenants saying that they would be prepared to pay £1,100 of the money they owed us...hooray! It was short £100 but neither Dave nor I could cope with the stress of trying to squeeze that out of them.

We popped out to buy Dave's mum, Janet, a birthday card and a cool sparkler shaped as a 70 for the cake we were going to pick up on Saturday.

It was back to the D.I.Y. when we got in as we made a start on stripping out the old kitchen ready for the new one. Soon the car was full of broken cupboards and flaky lino. I cooked a lovely Chinese dinner on the camping stove and we crashed out for the night.

Thursday 13th March

I had period-like pains on and off all day today and felt exhausted. I thought of getting a doctor's appointment to check it wasn't a urinary tract infection. While I lay on the sofa Dave painted the kitchen ceiling. We had Chinese again and later as Dave joined me on the sofa I felt Pear moving around. It was so exciting; Dave and I spent ages with our hands on my tummy waiting for him to wiggle.

Friday 14th March

Today was Janet's birthday, so we telephoned her and sang a very out of tune Happy Birthday to her.

The postman delivered a letter from our agents saying that the freeholder had decided to put our freehold up for auction and of all the days they had to pick it landed on Pear's due date! I filed it in the pile I've called, 'Let's worry about that another day!'

I went to the doctor's to get my urine checked out and it was clear which was good. My blood test results had also come back fine, although I was at the low end of the iron deficiency scale - which explained why I had been so tired recently. We went to Infinity Foods and stocked up on loads of iron-rich foods for lunch and dinner. I was feeling a lot happier now that Pear was moving around quite a bit, it was very comforting.

In the evening Dave went on the BabyCentre website and we had such a giggle testing ourselves on how many nursery rhymes we knew. I did marginally better than Dave but realised that I had changed the words to many of them, including 'The Grand Old Duke of York' - which I sung, had 5 thousand men and Dave asked where the other 5 thousand had got to? We needed to swot up before Pear arrived.

Saturday 15th March

While Dave was on another long run I got one of my super addictive Infinity Cafe salads and took it to the beach. It was quite warm so I relaxed for a bit before going for a wander. Dave and I picked up a delicious looking chocolate cake for Janet's surprise birthday meal tomorrow. We had splashed out on a vegan version so my sister-in-law, Karen and I - who are both vegan - could join in with the cake eating festivities.

After the meal we were planning on driving to our house in London to see what condition the dreaded 'guinea-pig' tenants had left it in and fix anything that needed repairing before re-letting it. Dave's brother Doug and Karen had also said they would pay Dave to do some work on a flat they own nearby, which was great as we definitely could do with the extra cash, but also hard because it would take us away from all the things that needed doing in Brighton.

It was ridiculous how much stuff we ended up packing in the car. As well as my old friend - Mr Inflatable Bed - we had a duvet, pillows, Dave's tools and even a step ladder. The car was so packed there wasn't anywhere to put Janet's cake. We decided that it would melt, or I would eat it if it was left on my lap so in the end Dave wedged it on the top rung of the ladder right in front of the air-conditioning - it wafted tantalising chocolate fumes at us the entire journey.

The traffic was horrendous so instead of meeting Doug and Karen at their house at 12 pm we had to drive straight to the restaurant and made it there with minutes to spare before the agreed time of 1 pm. Janet was over the moon to see everyone and we had such a lovely meal and family catch-up. We told everyone our news that Pear was a boy and Doug cracked me up when he just couldn't stop looking at my baby bump. After the meal we went back to Doug and Karen's where we gave

Janet her joint pressie from the 4 of us - a Fortnum and Mason picnic hamper. She and Tony left for home at 6 pm and we had been planning on heading off too until I got a horrible stomach ache and nearly threw up - most likely a mixture of stress from the drive, baby and too much cake. Doug and Karen suggested we stay over which we decided to take them up on as I really didn't fancy getting to our London house late; especially if it was in a bad state as I definitely had no energy for cleaning.

Monday 17th March

We were all up at the ungodly hour of 6.30 am as Doug was keen to get an early start on the flat, Yuk! I just wanted to stay snuggled up in bed. Dave and I drove straight to our house and thankfully it wasn't too bad, there were some scratches on what had been new laminate flooring in the hallway and the place smelt really doggie but everything else appeared OK.

We dumped our belongings off and drove to Doug and Karen's flat to meet them. While Dave and Doug got started on the bathroom Karen and I went to buy some parking permits for Dave to use during the week. What a nightmare, it took so long and once we had eventually got some, we got stuck driving round and round the car park searching for the exit. While we were beginning to think we would be there forever I got a phone call from the guy at the inventory company saying he was waiting for me at the house. We managed to find the exit and made it over before he left. He was a bit of a wind-up to begin with making me feel like I was being picky about the scratches on the floor. We had also noticed that paint had been spilt on the bedroom carpet and he tried saying it was just 'wear and tear'. He did, however, start to see my point when I showed him the decking the tenants had constructed in the garden that was decidedly dangerous looking. He agreed it would need taking up before a new tenant moved in as they might hurt themselves on it and said we could bill the tenants for the disposal of it. Personally I couldn't see how we would get anymore money out of them.

After he had left I did some laundry and went to hang it up in the garden. As I looked out the kitchen window I couldn't see the washing line that usually hung between our pear tree and a 6 ft concrete pole. I figured the tenants must have taken it down for some strange reason. When I got outside I was gobsmacked to see that the pole was gone, and even more staggeringly, so was our horse-chestnut tree! I just couldn't believe that someone would go to the effort to remove a reinforced concrete pole and a tree especially in someone else's property. I sat down for a bit, in shock and then I felt quite cross all over again with the inventory company. They had boasted in their paperwork that the tenants had re-potted a plant in the hallway and yet they had managed to overlook something as big as an entire missing tree! As my dad would say - it beggared belief.

Tuesday 18th March

I woke up with a terribly sore throat - I wondered if I got it from ranting at the inventory guy?

My friend Emma came to visit with Connor who is now 3 months old and even more gorgeous than the last time I saw him, if that was possible. We had a good old gossip and I grilled her on all aspects of being a mummy. She seemed to be doing so well and certainly didn't look like she'd had a baby just a few months ago; I hoped I could get back in shape as quickly.

Later on as I was busy cooking a stew ready for when Dave got in, our letting agent and new tenants turned up unannounced to measure up. It was a good job I'd tidied up as I always like to start a tenancy by creating a good impression with a clean property. The couple seemed nice enough and asked if they could paint one of the bedrooms that the previous tenants had, in a moment of sheer lunacy - probably shortly after they pulled up our tree - painted purple! I said it should be OK as long as they promised to keep it neutral.

Tips & things to do

- Your baby's body is now covered in 'lanugo' which is a very fine hair.

- If your baby gets hiccups you may be able to feel it.

- Many of the pregnancy books say that this part of your pregnancy is a good time to go away on holiday as most of the more unpleasant pregnancy symptoms have passed and you are still not too big to feel uncomfortable travelling.

- You may find your skin feels a bit itchy on your tummy as it continues to stretch to accommodate your growing baby. Keep using a good moisturiser or oil and drink lots of water.

- Try to find time everyday to put your feet up and relax.

Will I ever reach
the blooming stage?

Wednesday 19th March

Another friend, Richard from my old workplace, popped by today for a quick catch up and afterwards dropped me off at Emma's for lunch. We played with Connor; he is so cute, it was a good job I was already pregnant as being with him had made me decidedly broody!

After lunch Emma needed to change something at Mamas and Papas so I went along for the ride. It was full of lots of lovely things, I was incredibly restrained making just one tiny purchase, a pair of white baby socks with 'Welcome to the World' written in blue - absolutely gorgeous.

Thursday 20th March

While Dave was slogging away again at Doug and Karen's bathroom I went to see my lovely osteopath, Donald, for a treatment. He was so pleased with the news of my pregnancy but did bring me down to earth a bit when he commented that my legs were looking veiny and that I should do some exercise. I had been quite precious with this pregnancy - as I just hadn't wanted to do anything to chance losing our baby - but I guessed I was at a point where things should be OK and a bit of gentle exercise might be beneficial after all.

Friday 21st March

My sore throat had gone, replaced by a bunged up nose and headache. I vacuumed the house with a Hoover the tenants had left. I soon realised why they hadn't taken it when the entire house was filled with a strong doggie odour.

Pear had been keeping me excellent company all day; every time I called his name he kicked me, bless him - how clever!

Saturday 22nd March

I had planned on taking a trip into central London today, but the weather was so wet and yucky it seemed daft to go risking getting a worse cold than I already had. Instead I did some more cleaning - tenants don't you just love them! All I wanted was to feel better, get home to Brighton and for the weather to improve, was that too much to ask? Donald's comments about the veins in my legs had made me paranoid so I forced myself do a bit of exercise. Well I walked around the living room 100 times and did some gentle leg exercises then called it a day as I was feeling rough again. I took to bed - one good thing was that the tenants left a bed, but I was trying not to think too hard as to whether their dogs had slept on it! At least we weren't on our inflatable mattress. My head was aching so much I just lay there, couldn't even face reading or watching telly.

Sunday 23rd March

Dave was scheduled to go on a 20 mile run today; he got up early to go and then discovered it was snowing, unbelievable in March!

Eventually the snow turned to rain and despite my saying he was crazy to go out in such foul weather, Dave set off for his mammoth run. He was gone 4 hours and when he returned I massaged his cold, aching calf muscles. My head still hurt when I bent forward and later as we snuggled in bed - you've guessed it - my horrible tummy ache returned. As I wriggled around crying in pain it made me wonder how I would cope with giving birth when a stomach ache could get me so badly. I succumbed once again to some Gaviscon and it eased off.

Monday 24th March

I woke up at 8 am with such a dry mouth and I felt so hot; the heating had kicked in overnight making me feel like a boil-in-the-bag ready-meal. We opened the windows to let some fresh air in; I blew my nose and ended up making it bleed...Yuk!

I wondered when I would start experiencing the wonderful phenomena I kept reading about, the blooming part of pregnancy - I just felt blooming terrible!

Dave was chivvying me along as I'd asked if we could go to the supermarket before he went to Doug's flat; one thing I certainly didn't miss was living somewhere where everything involved a car ride. I felt quite tearful as I was still feeling ropey and would rather be in bed, but knew if we didn't go to the store I would be alone all day with no food.

I felt better once the fridge was filled with lots of healthy stuff to tide us over until we got home. The bathroom at Doug and Karen's flat was taking longer than expected - as was the case with all D.I.Y. ventures I'd come across to date. Today was no exception as when the bath was delivered it was damaged and so Dave wasted loads of time getting a replacement.

Tuesday 25th March

The day started well with Dave making time for a kiss and a cuddle before heading off to the flat for another day's graft. It was nice because he had been leaving so early most mornings that I hadn't seen him till the evenings when I was really not at my best!

I spent some time tidying up the garden, quite frustrating though, if I wasn't pregnant I would have had a go at dismantling the dodgy decking myself, but I decided it was probably best not to risk it. I got so carried away; I left it too late to eat as it was gone 2 pm by the time I got in. My stomach started aching so I lay down for a while then had a soak in the bath for nearly an hour. By the time I got out I felt much better until I had dinner and back came the pains again - twice in one day seemed so unfair! I felt particularly tearful and sorry for myself.

Tips & things to do

- Your baby can hear your voice and also your heartbeat. So talk and sing to him or her throughout the day.

- Your baby's lungs are continuing to mature and he or she probably weighs about half a pound by now.

- If you brush your teeth too vigorously or blow your nose hard - as I did -you may notice some bleeding as the blood supply increases in your body.

- To help combat getting restless legs and varicose veins take some gentle exercise at least 3 times a week.

- Try to graze continually throughout the day with healthy little snacks rather than eating 3 big meals, I found it difficult to change my eating habits and suffered with indigestion and stomach ache throughout my entire pregnancy.

Lots to do...

Wednesday 26th March

Dave went to the flat to finish a few bits and pieces off. He did promise he would be done by 12 pm, but as is usual in D.I.Y. - land it was 2 pm by the time he finally downed tools. It took him ages to clear the, condemned - by us - decking in the garden and 3 trips to the tip to get rid of the rubbish. I felt so bad not to be helping him more as he lugged planks of wood past me, but he insisted I let him do it. Instead I cleaned the house to within an inch of its life and soon it was sparkling from top to bottom; I wondered how long that would last.

We eventually got home at 9.45 pm, tired but so happy to be back in Brighton and our lovely little flat.

Thursday 27th March

Today was spent catching up on boring paperwork, filing and phone calls to give meter readings from our London house to the gas and electricity companies. Hopefully I had read them correctly as I did give myself a bit of an unpleasant surprise a while back when I gave them too many digits and we ended up with a £3,000 bill...gulp!

Dave had been walking round like a zombie all day exhausted from all the D.I.Y. at Doug and Karen's place. I hoped he recovered soon as I had a long list for him too!

In the afternoon we went for my appointment with a midwife called Ruth. She was lovely to us, answering all our questions and indulging me in my favourite bit - hearing Pear's little heart beat. I noticed on the shelf behind her that she had several very realistic models of babies. I asked to see the one most similar to Pear in size - making her and Dave laugh as I held it up to my tummy trying to imagine that I really had a baby in there. Dave and I were buzzing as we left, seeing the model and how big and perfect it looked got us extremely excited. For probably the first time we started making plans for Pear's arrival, we joked about what things he may like - Dave thought motorbikes, I thought power tools, after all he had spent his entire life so far listening to Black and Decker drills etc!

Saturday 29th March

We had a busy day today; since we'd been back the realisation of how much work needed doing on the Brighton place had started to sink in. We popped out for a bit of fresh air - as the sun was shining - before Dave made a start on drilling holes for the new electrics in the kitchen. I cleared the hallway that was chokka full of boxes and bags of goodness knows what!

Our friends Nick and Catherine rang to say they were in the area and would like to come and see us, which prompted a further burst of cleaning in the bathroom. We were storing a chest of drawers and dissembled wardrobe there so you couldn't even shut the bathroom door.

When they arrived they seemed quite surprised to see how we were living. As they were greeted by me and my bump happily cooking away on a camping stove precariously balanced on a chair in a 'living room' so piled up with clutter that it would be hard for even the tiniest of people to actually 'live in'!

Not surprisingly we decided to eat out and Nick treated us all to a lovely meal at our local veggie pub, The George. It was great catching up with them both and they even offered to come back in a few weeks time to help us get on top of things...Yay, thank goodness for wonderful friends!

I didn't feel Pear moving as much today - either because we were so busy or maybe he was feeling shy as we had guests!

Monday 31st March

I sorted out some paperwork today and tried to work my way through a 'things to do' list. A tricky task as no sooner had I crossed something off it then another thing replaced it.

Dave was still doing 'prep' work in the kitchen - channelling out the wall to make way for the wiring for the new electric cooker and extractor hood we planned on getting. I am not very patient at the beginning stages of a project - preferring the finishing touches like painting, rather than all the unseen graft that takes ages but doesn't look at the end of the day as though you have much to show for your labours.

I nipped out to buy ingredients to make a Chinese stir fry - as it was easy to cook on our camping stove and seemed to be one of the few things that didn't give me indigestion.

Tips & things to do

- As your bump grows you may have backache or puffy ankles, try to put your feet up several times during the day. If your back is aching you could book an appointment to see an Osteopath.

- Your baby is looking more like a baby now; hair continues to grow and the eyelashes and eyebrows start to form.

- This week if your baby were to be born he or she would have a reasonable chance of survival with specialist care.

- See if there is any pregnancy yoga or antenatal swimming classes you could attend in your area.

- Take some time-out to catch up with friends and your partner. Once your baby arrives you will want to spend all your time with him or her.

Pregnancy yoga class...

Wednesday 2nd April

I had such a great nights sleep last night and woke up feeling refreshed. I went to my first pregnancy yoga class - handily just a few streets away. There was only me and one other lady but I really enjoyed it and couldn't think of a more pleasant way to spend an hour and a half relaxing and gently stretching my body.

When I got home I was rewarded for holding on the phone for absolutely ages to the Citizens Advice Bureau, by being told I should receive something called Maternity Allowance. I qualified for it from my old job, as I had worked within the specified time-frame. It was great news as although I had managed to save a bit of money it wouldn't be long before we would need to buy a pushchair, car seat and crib.

Thursday 3rd April

I felt a bit spaced out all day, maybe because the weather had taken a turn for the warmer. I went to the beach for some fresh air and what was becoming my almost daily ritual; an Infinity Food salad.

When I got back in Dave had papered the chimney breast in the kitchen and removed the last of the units, which meant we had no kitchen sink.

We placed an order for some gorgeous granite worktop that I had been drooling over for as long as I could remember. It was black with silver sparkly bits running through it, I joked with Dave that it was a fairy-dust worktop but fortunately that didn't put him off. Even though the flat was tiny and certainly a far cry from a family house like our London and Dover properties we had decided to make it as lovely as we could. It had been so many years now where all our D.I.Y. had been aimed towards tenants - dare I say magnolia paint and maple kitchen units. Three of our properties even had the same beige bathroom tiles because they were cheap and easy to stick up. I couldn't explain the happiness I felt when I lay in bed looking at the beautiful 'Pavilion' wallpaper my mum put up for us and hopefully the worktop would inspire the same level of joy - although at this very moment I would have plumped for any kitchen with a sink!

In the evening I got indigestion again and at one point actually thought I was going to be sick, but thankfully I wasn't. Pear wasn't very active today which made me worry about him.

Saturday 5th April

Yesterday as the weather was so lovely Dave and I played hooky and instead of working on the flat went to the beach. It always made me feel as if I was being naughty if I cut loose when there was work to be done, but we really needed some quality relaxation time together.

Last night I slept so well - probably as a result of the chilled out day we had - no tummy ache for a change, yippee!

We went to a local laundrette as neither of us had many clean clothes left to wear. It was amazing how much it cost, especially as we used the dryer as well and now all our clothes had a slightly scorched aroma!

Pear was reassuringly active today, bumping around happily. Dave and I ate at Wagamama in the evening; I had an enormous bowl of soup that kept me up weeing all night.

Sunday 6th April

I managed to lay-in until 11 am today which was wonderful - I loved our bedroom!

When I looked out the window I was amazed after yesterday's sunshine to see it had snowed in the night. Dave and I grabbed the camera and our coats and headed to The Pavilion to take some pictures of it dressed in snow and looking very pretty. We cracked up when we saw a group of teenagers had made a snowman complete with huge willy doing something unmentionable to a snow lady! We hung around eavesdropping as a couple of burly Pavilion security guards tried not to laugh as they asked the youths if they could remove the offending appendage - which they duly did.

Pear was particularly active all day, I'd taken to describing it as him 'moving furniture' around inside me. In the evening as I lay in the bath he moved, what looked to me like a mini grand piano, from one side of my tummy to the other! I shrieked out to Dave to come and look, as up until now we had only felt him when our hands were on my stomach. The pair of us - or should

I say 3 of us - played 'moving furniture' for ages, until Pear decided he had indulged us enough for one day.

Tuesday 8th April

All the snow magically vanished in the night and it was a lovely sunny day.

The kitchen had turned into what in the trade was referred to as 'a can of worms'. Now that the lino was gone it had revealed floorboards that were all rotten and needed replacing. The extra time spent fixing that and sorting out the gas and electrics would put our schedule back a bit...Hey ho what could you do?

I had started to feel a lot better; I was walking every day, doing some gentle exercises morning and night and even doing my pelvic floor exercises. If there was a prize to be given I thought I should definitely receive a gold star for effort!

Tips & things to do

- Keep up your pelvic floor exercises - trust me you will be glad I nagged you about them someday!

- Your baby will continue to gain weight, making him or her appear less wrinkled and their eyes may open for the first time around now.

- Your uterus reaches halfway between your navel and your sternum.

- If you haven't done so already look into what Maternity rights you have. The Citizens Advice Bureau is great for answering any questions you may have and pregnancy magazines are a good source of info on this subject.

Hunger pains...

Friday 11th April

The last couple of days were brilliant, no tummy ache which left me feeling great. I'd been finding that where we'd been eating earlier in the evening that instead of getting indigestion I was waking up anytime between 1 am and 3 am with hunger pains instead! I solved that little dilemma by sneaking upstairs while Dave slept and ate some fruity soya yoghurt. Dave thought it was quite funny and could tell the level of my hunger pains by how many empty pots he found in the morning on the sofa - my record so far was 3.

While Dave carried on with the kitchen renovations I nipped to the Jog Shop to buy him a nice bright running shirt so he would be easier to spot at The London Marathon this weekend. I plumped for neon yellow and spent the afternoon cutting black fabric into the letters of his name and stitching them on the front. Later on we drove to London to stay with our friends Emma and Al in preparation for Dave's big run.

Sunday 13th April

Today Dave was up at 5 am to eat porridge before the run - I didn't join him! I went with Emma to the top of her road as it was usually a great place to see the runners pass by. Despite us keeping our eyes peeled we didn't spot Dave which was disappointing - to be fair it was just a sea of runners, that after a while of watching closely made my eyes go funny!

I walked to Woolwich and caught a train into London where I had lunch before meeting up with Doug and Karen. We made our way along Embankment to find a good viewpoint and luckily we were near a bridge as it absolutely chucked it down with rain. I was sure the runners were grateful for the cooling shower but we weren't! The crowds were about 3 deep all along the pavement but amazingly we spotted Dave and whether it was because I was pregnant or just looking wet and sorry for myself but the crowd parted allowing me to get to the front whereupon Dave ran over and kissed me...so lovely. He completed the race in 4 hrs 45 minutes which was great and he looked in pretty good shape at the end. We went to Charing Cross Hotel for tea and cake and for Doug to give Dave's calf muscles a good rub down. I was so tired - my theory about marathons, a bit like that age old fact that if you work in a cake shop you will put on weight even if you don't eat the cakes, was that if you watched enough people running past you that by the end of the day you too would feel as though you had run a marathon!

We decided to stay an extra night at Emma and Al's as both of us were exhausted and the long drive home would probably have finished Dave's leg muscles off completely.

Monday 14th April

Bit of a mad rush around in the morning as Emma needed to be somewhere early so it was all systems go for us to leave at the same time as her. We popped into Sainsbury's and then a cafe for beans on toast before driving home. As we still had no parking permit we parked about 20 minutes away from the flat and walked. I got very hot and hungry and as soon as we got in I wolfed down a sandwich and ended up with stomach ache for my haste. I lay in the bath, crying in pain and feeling pathetic...oh dear!

Tips and things to do

- Your baby is sensitive to light now if you were to shine a torch at your tummy he or she may move their head towards the light. Dave and I had fun playing this little game but Pear had other ideas, I think he was sleeping or ignoring us as I didn't feel him move.

- Your baby's heart is beating 120-160 beats per minute.

- You may feel sudden tightening then relaxing sensations in your uterus called 'Braxton Hicks'. This is your body's way of having a practice run.

Finally I find a bra…

Wednesday 16th April

We were up early as we both had dentist's appointments in London - that had to be top of my list of things to do, get a dentist in Brighton! My appointment went OK but as per usual I felt nervous and I didn't think Pear liked it either as he jumped around a lot, especially when the dentist turned the drill on.

Afterwards we went to Bluewater for some calming retail therapy and pizza. I found the bra store Rigby and Peller which is apparently the bra company the Queen uses. I got fitted for a bra and it felt so much more comfortable than the one I'd been wearing - a bit of a royal price at nearly £50 but I was desperate for a bra that fitted me and I could say without hesitation that I had hunted everywhere else. I also found a fabulous pair of maternity jeans in 'Blooming Marvellous'. Up until now I had been resisting the urge to wear jeans as I couldn't bear anything tight near my tummy, but as I was getting bigger by the day even my tracksuit bottoms felt uncomfortable with me unable to decide whether to tie them above or below my bump. The first pair of jeans I tried on was amazingly comfy, they had a big soft fabric waistband that could either be folded to sit at your waist or opened to cover your entire tummy. As I pulled them over my bump it felt so nice not having buttons, zips or elastic digging in anywhere - wished I had discovered them sooner!

Before driving home Dave and I went into John Lewis to look at pushchairs. Oh my goodness, there were so many choices. One of the sales assistants gave us a demo of a few different styles and I had a little drive of one but succeeded in running Dave over and getting stuck behind a display...whoops, I was going to need to get some practice in! After about 45 minutes Dave and I were both feeling pretty flustered and spaced out. We decided to do some research and ask Emma how her pushchair performed before making our minds up. Dave was so sweet his only criteria being that it was a 3 wheeler so he could take Pear running with him...bless!

Thursday 17th April

Poor Dave felt ill today. We weren't sure if was flu, food poisoning, or the after effects of the marathon. I persuaded him to lie down while I went out to get a salad for lunch for me and soup for him if he felt up to it later.

The rest of the day I cleaned, tidied and played 'Florence Nightingale' while Dave rested. It made a change for it to be me looking after him as it was usually the other way round. Pear kept me great company today; moving furniture around his tiny home and sticking what Dave had jokingly referred to as a 'Black and Decker' out every now and then. I loved it when he was active as it felt so reassuring; many of my books said that as he got bigger I might feel fewer movements so I planned to enjoy them.

Friday 18th April

I slept so well last night but Dave was still feeling rough today with a choppy stomach. I was hoping I didn't get it as I had just started feeling good. I had a relaxing bath and lunch before going to Aveda for a free facial. It was so nice getting pampered - I couldn't remember the last time I had a facial. I did end up spending quite a bit of money on products to use at home though.

In the evening I felt terrible and threw up, which was a first - and with any luck last - in my pregnancy.

Sunday 20th April

I felt absolutely fine today despite being sick the other night and Dave was back on form as well.

We walked to the park and had a bit of an impromptu picnic on a bench as it was such a lovely, sunny day. Later we made a trip to the tip to get rid of all the kitchen debris we had accumulated. The car was bursting at the seams and every time Dave braked a bit of kitchen unit bashed me on the head.

Tuesday 22nd April

I didn't sleep great last night - a combination of an over-active mind and Pear practicing gymnastics by the feel of it.

We had quite a busy day as we needed to take the car to the Volvo garage as it was making a strange noise and attracting funny looks from pedestrians!

The day whizzed by and we decided to eat out in the evening as I wasn't feeling inspired as to what to cook/heat-up on our camping stove. I was so hungry I stuffed myself silly in The George pub - hoping I wouldn't regret that later!

Tips and things to do

- At the end of this week you will have finished the 2nd trimester...hooray!

- Take some time to pamper yourself with a facial or whatever makes you feel good.

- This week your baby's eyelids begin to open and his or her retinas will start to form.

- Be prepared that you may need to purchase several bras during your pregnancy to accommodate your ever changing boob size. I was a total novice at this and found it all a bit of an alien concept as I had been wearing the same size bra for years. I did amuse a sales assistant when she noticed I was wearing a nursing bra quite early on in my pregnancy. It was the only one that fit me at the time and I had naively thought it would see me through my pregnancy and breastfeeding. I now know that it is far better to buy bras as and when you feel you need them rather than stock-piling lots of the same size.

- Treating yourself to some maternity wear is a must. I thought I could make do with my wardrobe of assorted Lycra tops and trackkie bottoms but many of them became uncomfortable as my bump grew. Maternity wear is cut to ensure a comfy fit and yet the hemlines will all still hang well to flatter your lovely baby bump. My 'Blooming Marvellous' maternity jeans were exactly that - blooming marvellous! My only regret was that I didn't buy them sooner.

- Around this time you may be offered a glucose tolerance test by your midwife. She will be checking your blood sugar levels to make sure you don't have gestational diabetes. This is a type of diabetes that some women get during pregnancy that usually goes once your baby has been born.

WEEK 28 – THE 3rd TRIMESTER

We get by with a little help from our friends...

Wednesday 23rd April

I went for my pregnancy yoga class today - it was funny, I thought that being a dancer I would be quite good at yoga but not so! Yoga seemed to use a totally different set of muscles to my ballet trained ones. At least I wouldn't get bored in class as I tried to master the squat and the downward hare or upward dog - whatever they might be!

Dave was onto the kitchen floor at last so we thought we might finally be turning a corner but then we ran out of under-lay half-way across the room. As it was a nice evening we walked up to Screwfix to order some more to be delivered tomorrow and spent the rest the evening watching TV.

Thursday 24th April

We were up early today as I had an appointment with the midwife. I made the decision not to take the glucose test as it involved drinking quite a bit of Lucozade and when I read the label on the bottle it was full of caffeine, which with my body being the temple it is - ha, would probably not be a great idea. I used to make everyone laugh at work when I was bouncing off the walls after drinking organic cola, plus Pear jumped around if I ate just a couple of squares of dark chocolate, so the two of us would be hyper for hours. The midwife was great and said she would still be able to test me by taking a blood and urine sample so everyone was happy. I told her that I had been a bit worried about my size as a few people (mostly total strangers might I add) had commented on how small I was. She measured my bump and said I was the perfect size for the stage I was at which was a huge relief - note to self, ignore people who don't know what they are talking about!

Friday 25th April

Our lovely friends Nick and Catherine came to stay to help us with the kitchen... a big hooray for fabulous friends!

While the boys went to pick up the kitchen units Catherine did a bath full of washing-up for us - refusing my offers of help, bless her. I cooked us all a fry-up on the camping-stove and once we had chowed that down we admired the units that looked even better than I remembered them from the showroom.

The day went so quickly and before we knew it our tummies - mine especially - were rumbling for dinner. We ate at the pub and had a good catch up with each other as we hadn't had much of a chance during the day. Nick had been a hard taskmaster in the kitchen refusing offers of tea and coffee for both him and Dave with a polite, 'No thanks Charlie, we've got to get on'. Brilliant, just the kick up the bottom we both needed, I could see more progress was going to happen in a few days than in the last few weeks.

Somehow we managed to make enough space in the living room for Nick and Catherine to sleep on our blow-up mattress. Catherine had vowed to help me clear some of the clutter the next day, she was going to need to perform magic tricks to do that as I wasn't sure where we could clear it to - oh to have a garage!

Saturday 26th April

I slept well last night; my stomach did ache a bit but it was more a feeling of my ligaments stretching than actual tummy ache.

After breakfast the boys set up camp in the kitchen and Catherine and I started sorting through boxes and boxes of stuff in the living room. Every time I went past the kitchen another unit had been attached to the wall which was so exciting. Catherine sorted through all our kitchen bits and pieces and whenever the boys went downstairs to cut up wood we snuck into the kitchen and started filling the units with food and crockery - until we got caught and banished back into our room that was! It was amazing how much space we created in the living room by moving the things that belonged in the kitchen into the units. It meant we were able to go through more boxes - well Catherine did; she insisted I watched her from the sofa and instructed her as to anything she could throw away. Where we had been living with minimal things for so long it was quite easy to say bye-bye to lots of useless clutter we had been storing.

Later we went for a wander around the local reclamation yard, but resisted the urge to purchase anything - after feeling so good about clearing our excess junk it would be crazy to replace it with more. We bought ourselves salads and brought back some veggie burgers for the boys who practically had to be wrestled with to get them to down tools! The fitter turned up to measure the space for our new sparkly worktop. He did worry me a bit when he said that they would need a parking space at the front of the flat and an electricity supply when they came to fit it. That was going to be tricky as directly outside our flat the parking was disabled only and a motorbike bay - I decided to worry about that another time.

It was 9.30 pm by the time the boys had finally run out of steam and food, so we all headed off to Wagamama for a late supper.

Sunday 27th April

Dave and Nick went to our car to get a TV set my Aunty had kindly given us. It was absolutely massive, most definitely a two man job, that or a hernia waiting to happen!

Catherine and I went on a hunt for French pastries for breakfast - we had worked out that the quality of food was reflected in the work taking place in the kitchen, which so far was top notch!

It was such a productive day, the kitchen units were all in and the boys cut the entire plinth to go around the bottom of the units. We decided against using the wraps we had bought as it looked perfect as it was. If we took them back to the store we would get the money back on them - £422 not to be sniffed at.

While the boys finished up in the kitchen Catherine and I completed clearing the living room - it was great to be able to see the floor again albeit covered in carpet that had seen better days.

Dave and I managed to persuade Nick and Catherine to let us take them out for dinner as they had been treating us ever since they arrived. We had a delicious meal at Terre à Terre and returned home for a final blitz of the flat. Between Dave and Nick they managed to heave my 2 old trunks from boarding school days that were packed full of costumes into the loft. Then with Catherine's help the 3 of them formed a chain passing my 'treasures' down to me that I had been desperate to be reunited with. It was like Christmas as I sat on the kitchen floor unwrapping the bubble wrap from our beautiful wedding china and finally putting it all away in the kitchen cupboards.

It was 9.30 pm by the time the last piece of china had been safely deposited in its new home and we said our goodbyes to Nick and Catherine. It was hard to put into words just how grateful we were to them for all their help but I thought they got the message. We had been feeling so snowed under with the seemingly never-ending amount of work needing doing before Pear made his entrance, but at least now we were a step closer to having a home ready in time for him.

Tuesday 29th April

I had been sleeping like a log since the weekend; all the activity and excitement at seeing things' getting done had exhausted me. Yesterday Dave and I were both so tired that we even ended up napping in the afternoon - we hoped we hadn't worn Nick and Catherine out as much as they had to return to work after grafting for us.

I slept in today until 10 am, lovely! I spent a few hours sorting out paperwork before nipping to Laura Ashley to pick up some wallpaper samples. Catherine had come up with a great idea of covering the spines of all our ratty looking files with wallpaper as they would eventually be placed on shelves in the living room and would blend in better. I also made a quick stop at Montezuma's chocolate shop to buy Nick and Catherine some goodies as a thank you.

Tips and things to do

- Your baby's eyelids and lashes are now present and the hair on his or her head starts growing.

- You may experience leg cramps, haemorrhoids, varicose veins, itchy skin, swelling and indigestion! But if you are anything like me all these negatives will be outweighed by the growing excitement at having reached the final stretch known as the 3rd Trimester.

- If your partner is working he may want to look into what paternity leave he is entitled to.

- You may want to find out about childbirth classes in your area.

- If friends or family offer their services make the most of it especially if like us you are still a long way off being ready.

We celebrate our wedding anniversary, on the wrong day...

Wednesday 30th April

Nick came over to help Dave for a few hours today after he had dropped Catherine off at Gatwick where she was working for the day.

As I left for my yoga class the washing-machine and fridge arrived, complete with a grumpy man who said he wouldn't carry them up the stairs; even though I had explained when I booked it that we lived in an upside-down house. It was so lucky for us that Nick chose today to come round as Dave would never have managed alone. I left them to it and spent the next hour and half relaxing or at least trying to. Dom, my yoga teacher, might well be a mind-reader as when we were doing a relaxation exercise she instructed us to clear our minds and not to think about what we were having for dinner just as I was doing exactly that! I thought that learning how to switch off would be so beneficial for me; if I could ever master it as my brain always seemed to be ticking away. Afterwards I went for tea with one of the other girls from the class, called Cheryl, which was really nice. She was just one week behind me in her pregnancy so we could hopefully keep each other company. One of my biggest wishes upon moving to Brighton was to make new friends so I was well on my way.

When I got home the washing-machine and fridge were both fitted in the kitchen and looked amazing - we'd chosen to get both appliances in black to blend with the worktop and 2 of the wall units which had a high gloss, black finish to them. The only casualty had been the wall on the stairway where a big gouge had been left by the grumpy guy (well the washing-machine to be precise) no doubt he was making a silent protest at having to help lug the things up the stairs. Dave and Nick had also found time to fit the extractor hood over the hob so the kitchen was coming together at last.

Thursday 1st May

Dave made a bit of a discovery today when he realised that between the kitchen designer, worktop fitter and us, we had over-looked two quite big details. As the kitchen currently was laid out, once the granite worktop was fitted the first glitch was that we wouldn't be able to open the soap drawer on the washing-machine and even more worryingly, the washing-machine would be stuck there forever…whoops! Dave had to take out all the units he and Nick had spent so long fitting and trimmed about 6cm off each one before re-fitting it all, hopefully erasing our problems in the process. Unbelievably we had managed in just 2 days to do 5 wash loads of laundry, a personal record!

Friday 2nd May

I finally had a hairdresser's appointment today; it had been such a long time since my hair was last highlighted that it was a surprise seeing it looking nice for a change. Pear was pretty active the entire appointment - most likely because I was sitting down with nothing to distract myself with so I was more aware of him bouncing around on the trampoline he had in there!

Saturday 3rd May

I felt great today sporting my freshly done hair and wearing a pink jumper I discovered in the loft that made my bump look fabulous.

Dave made a start on putting up some shelves in the living room so we could free up more floor space. We were trying to save money and had decided to use the wood from our IKEA wardrobes to build them. It did seem a bit rash taking a saw to them but there was absolutely no room to assemble them and we already had a large built-in wardrobe and cupboard space in the bedroom. The wardrobes were slightly worse for wear anyway, they certainly had seen a few places; they started off in our house in London, moved to Folkestone, then to Dover before getting here so we had got some good use out of them. Making them into shelves had to be the ultimate way to recycle them.

While Dave was being a 'handy Andy' I went to buy him an anniversary card and pressie. I got him the most enormous bar of chocolate from Montezuma's - it was coconut and macadamia nuts and was a kilo in weight so it should last him a while.

When I got in Dave had finished the shelves in one alcove which I instantly filled with files and photo albums. We then went a little crazy taking up the manky carpet and underlay ready to put the laminate flooring down. We tumbled into bed absolutely exhausted but happy with the progress we had made.

Monday 5th May

Dave and I celebrated our wedding anniversary today. After exchanging cards and chocolate Dave put our wedding photos on the computer to watch while we got ready. We dumped the carpet off at the tip and spent a couple of hours relaxing on the beach before coming home to make a start on wallpapering one of the walls in the living room. We stayed up late doing it, I was chief cutter as it was another patterned paper from Laura Ashley and this time I didn't make the mistakes I did with the bedroom one. It went up pretty well although it was quite late by the time we finished so it was difficult to see the finished effect.

Tuesday 6th may

What a pair Dave and I are, we realised that today was actually our anniversary - and there we were telling our family as they rang to congratulate us that they had the wrong day! In our defence I think we got muddled because we were married in Vegas and they put the month and the day round the other way to us and that caused confusion at the time.

We made a start on laminating the floor in the living room but didn't make a huge amount of progress as there was a tricky piece by the doorway that needed lots of cutting.

Tips and things to do

- Getting your hair done can be such a boost around now, especially if like me you have neglected it for a long time!

- Your baby's head is now more in proportion to its body; and fat continues to accumulate on his or her body.

- Your baby is sensitive to light, sound, taste and smell. I felt little Pear jumping around whenever a siren went off in the street or when Dave started drilling.

- It is nice to start reading or singing to your baby around now. It can help you to bond with your baby and is relaxing - especially if you choose to give your vocal cords a flex in the bath.

- You may start to feel either impatient for the time to pass so you can meet your baby, or the total opposite - as I did - that you need more time to prepare.

Week 30

'We have to do it she's pregnant!'

Wednesday 7th May

In my pregnancy yoga class Dom asked us all to thank our babies for choosing us as their mum, which was a lovely notion and I liked to think that Pear chose us as his parents.

After my class Dave and I had lunch and spent the rest of the day laminating the living room floor - boy was it time consuming especially as I was on quality control and so many of the boards had been damaged.

Thursday 8th May

What a day! Dave was up at 6 am to get to Screwfix when it opened to buy a tap for the kitchen sink. It was nearly midnight last night when he suddenly realised that the worktop was getting fitted today and that the tap needed to go in before the worktop as it was solid granite; so once it was in it wouldn't be going anywhere!

The worktop fitters arrived at 7.45 am and were playing good guy, bad guy with me. One of them was like sunshine while the other had definitely got out of bed the wrong side and immediately started muttering about the lack of parking and our stairs. I did my best to look pathetic whilst trying to butter them up at the same time. Mr Miserable got on his mobile to head office and when he came off I heard him say to Mr Sunshine, 'We have to do it she's pregnant' - Nice one Pear!

It was a pretty stressful morning all in all - they didn't want to park their van far from our flat so they just left it in the disabled bay and asked me to keep an eye out for traffic wardens. I counted 9 in total pass by the top of our road and each time I found myself holding my breath hoping they wouldn't head down our street and miraculously they didn't. We made it through the morning with no parking tickets and the heavy granite worktops were fitted before we knew it. They looked amazing especially in the afternoon sun as the sparkly silver bits cast rainbow lights all over the kitchen walls. As the fitters packed away their tools even Mr Miserable managed to crack a smile when he saw how delighted I was with my lovely new kitchen.

Once they had gone Dave and I went on a mission to tidy up the mess they had left outside. There was dust and water everywhere and by the time we had finished we were both worn out. I got an early night and fell into a deep, deep sleep as I imagined did Pear. A bit later Dave came to bed and woke me up and poor Pear was so shocked he jumped and flipped around until my stomach started to ache. Dave felt really bad bless him.

Friday 9th May

Dave and I were on a mission today to try and finish the living room floor. Ideally we would have had an empty room to work with but we thought it would be easier to move the furniture around the room rather than clearing it - to be honest we didn't have much of a choice as there was nowhere to empty it too. Instead we found ourselves moving things as we progressed, the trickiest being the hernia TV set that in the end Dave put on a towel and we dragged it across the room. We finished the flooring and spent till 5 pm sweeping up the sawdust and arranging the TV and sofa where we wanted them. What a tiring but satisfying day it was.

Saturday 10th May

Dave and I had a bit of a mad morning. We whizzed to Howdens to change a kitchen unit door that was damaged, from there we went to the tip. I spotted a maternity wear store called 'Yummy Mummy Maternity' and we popped in there. I purchased a lovely white skirt with such a soft stretchy waistband that was going to be so useful if the weather remained sunny. We went a bit crazy in Sainsbury's buying so much frozen stuff - just because we could now we had our fabulous fridge-freezer. We had a quick lunch before another trip to Screwfix - we seemed to be living there nowadays. It was baking hot even at 4 pm so we sat outside a pub and had some cold drinks and a bit of a rest after our manic few hours.

Later we ate a delicious meal at Food for Friends where Dave reckoned he had the best sticky toffee pudding he had ever tasted - and we got pretty excited when Pear decided to entertain us with a few summersaults.

Sunday 11th May

It was another gorgeous day today - I love Brighton and I love it even more in the sun. I wore my new white skirt and roped Dave into bringing a few more of my things down from the loft. I would have liked to have gone up there myself but my bump was bit big now to be doing step ladders, plus I was not that good with height at the best of times. We went out for lunch and then later Dave went to Wickes while I started sorting through the boxes he had brought down for me. The highlight of the day was later on when I was laying in the bath and Pear stuck what I thought must have been his bottom right out. Then as I called out to Dave to come and see, this tiny hand or it could have been a foot shot out as well!

Tuesday 13th May

Yesterday our cooker was delivered so we now had a fully functioning kitchen...hooray! We had a bit of a nightmare today when Dave went to get the car and it wouldn't start. We were due at our dentist's in London in an hour and a half and knew we would end up having to pay a cancellation fee if we missed our appointments; so Dave got our old car insured for the day and we made it there just in time - phew!

After the dentist we went to see Emma and she gave me a bag full of baby clothes Connor has grown out of as well as some useful maternity wear for me. It was so exciting going through it all.

Tips and things to do

- Your baby weighs about 3 pounds now and his or her tiny toenails are starting to grow.

- Rather than hiding your bump in baggy clothes which will just make you feel fat why not show it off? I felt so proud of my growing bump and it certainly came in handy for getting our worktop fitters to cooperate!

- Making friends with other mums-to-be at this time is great; you will have someone else to chat to about your experiences who will understand what you're going through.

- Your baby may be quite active now and if there are any loud noises he or she may jump, like Pear did when Dave woke us both up. Sirens in the street also startled him and I found myself holding my tummy whenever a police car or ambulance whizzed by and saying words to comfort him.

- Keep up your pelvic floor exercises and practice squatting - my yoga teacher really emphasised how being able to do them would be helpful during our baby's birth and she was right.

Pear gets his first set of wheels!

Wednesday 14th May

I went to my yoga class while Dave called the RAC out to look at the car. I might have got a bit carried away with some of the stretches as later in the day my back started aching. Luckily the car was OK - just lacking in the petrol department...whoops!

We had a relaxing afternoon wandering around The Lanes and eating ice cream. After dinner I made a start on our joint account, not one of my favourite jobs at the best of times. I ended up feeling quite overwhelmed, firstly at the lack of funds in our account and then to top it off nicely I read an article about pregnancy online that said that many women had packed their hospital bags by now. I felt nowhere near ready and as I read the list of things they suggested you pack I found myself crying to Dave that I only had one thing on the list - a tube of toothpaste. Pear sensing my distress joined in by kicking me really hard, ouch!

Thursday 15th May

I had a lovely sleep last night despite getting myself in a bit of a state about things. My back was still aching from my yoga class - hopefully I hadn't done anything too serious to it.

Dave put some shelves up in our bedroom that I immediately filled with a few of our treasures. I loved our bedroom so much, it got more homely every day and I lay in bed for ages admiring the wallpaper - so it turned out to be excellent value for money. I spent the rest of the day washing all the baby clothes Emma gave us in a non-biological liquid ready for Pear.

Friday 16th May

I felt quite tearful today as Dave was being a bit grumpy with me for no apparent reason. I felt as though my body and my life were changing so much and I needed him to tell me how much he appreciated and loved me. I found myself praising him for everything he did especially all the D.I.Y. but today for some reason he was not being his usual loving self. I told him how I was feeling and he tried to reassure me that of course he loved me and noticed the little things I did around the place.

Later I went on a mission filing while Dave finished the shelves in the living room. We placed the rest of files on them, plus a few of my favourite books from the loft and it looked great.

Saturday 17th May

Dave and I ordered a bathroom today which was very exciting. We managed to negotiate a great price on a bath, toilet, 2 lovely units and a round ceramic basin as well as some gorgeous taps. It was going to be amazing owning a bathroom that wasn't from the trade range at Plumb Centre for a change.

I carried on with yesterday's filing and put labels on all the files, so I felt pretty impressed with myself. My tummy was particularly big tonight I was struggling to move around and once I sat on the floor I needed a winch or Dave to pull me up.

Sunday 18th May

I didn't sleep that well last night - a combination of trapped air from last nights Mexican food and Pear kicking me.

I got up at 10 am and tidied the kitchen, which was my pride and joy. Dave filled the car with yet more rubbish while I cleaned the kitchen and living room floors.

Later we met Dave's brother, John, at the seafront where he was with his Mini club. After having a good wander and look at all the cars we had dinner and a relaxing night for a change.

Monday 19th May

Dave and I dropped all the rubbish at the tip in the morning then drove to a lovely baby store near Portslade called 'Lili May', for a browse of pushchairs. We were leaning towards buying a 3 wheeler like Emma's as she seemed to think hers was pretty good. The assistant demonstrated the Quinny Buzz to us and it comes in a lovely midnight blue colour which we both liked. She did get me a bit worried when she explained that they only had one pushchair in stock and there was an 8 week wait to receive another. If Pear arrived on his due date we only had 9 weeks left so we needed to decide swiftly.

We had lunch together then popped to Screwfix to order yet more laminate flooring. I bought a lovely lampshade for the bedroom in a great shop nearby called Velvet. So we actually had one totally finished room, with the exception of a bit of trim that needed to go round the edge of the room where the laminate finished, Dave always liked to leave something to do for later!

We also ordered some great drawers for the bedroom as at the moment our clothes were all squished in the wardrobe - how I longed for a knickers and socks drawer, somewhere to balance my glass of water and other essential night-time nick-nacks. Pear was so active all day, even as I was walking around town, and in bed he kicked me loads... I loved it!

Tuesday 20th May

We managed to get out the house earlier than yesterday, stopping at the Volvo garage to pick up an iso-fix for the car seat we planned on buying. We went back to 'Lili May' and paid for the Quinny Travel System we test drove yesterday. It consisted of a pushchair called the Quinny Buzz that had 2 different sized liners to last until Pear was 4 years old and hopefully wouldn't need pushing anymore and a carry cot - rather sweetly named a 'Dreami' that Pear would be using until he could support his own head. There was also a Maxi-Cosi car seat that fitted onto the pushchair base for use if you were just planning on having your baby in it for 2 hours or less. I worked out that we made a £75 saving on the price of the 3 items from what I had seen in another baby store and we then saved a further £25 as the assistant gave us a store loyalty card - fantastic.

We had lunch and Dave spent a few hours cleaning our old Volvo ready to go on ebay. We set the Quinny pushchair up to check all the pieces were in the box and had a little play around - very exciting to have our first big baby purchase. It was funny, we probably spent more time and in some cases more money on Pear's first set of wheels than many of the cars we'd bought ourselves in the past!

Tips & things to do

- You may experience back ache as the weight from your ever increasing bump throws you off centre. Also as the ligaments in your body soften from all the pregnancy hormones it is easier to injure yourself - like my over-stretching in yoga class - so take it easy.

- Your stomach might start aching as your uterus stretches. It's now about 4 $\frac{1}{2}$ inches above your tummy.

- Your baby's brain is going through a stage of rapid development now.

- It is a good time to start thinking about the practical things you are going to need to purchase before your little one arrives. A car seat, pushchair and crib are all important items and looking into getting them now will be a big weight off your mind. We kept putting off buying anything as we just didn't want to tempt fate and then panicked that we had left it all too late.

- Try not to worry if you haven't organised anything at this point as there still is plenty of time and if your baby were to arrive early friends and family would rally round.

- If you do receive any baby clothes from friends take some time to wash them in a baby friendly non-biological washing powder and sort them into sizes ready for when you need them.

HypnoBirthing classes...

Wednesday 21st May

I did my yoga class in the morning which I enjoyed; I was getting the hang of this relaxing lark!

While Dave stripped the wallpaper in the bathroom I did yet more filing and then popped out to buy Pear some bits and pieces. I got him a couple of stripy, organic cotton bodysuits in 'JoJo Maman Bébé' and a swaddling blanket - as I read somewhere that after the confines of your tummy a baby likes to feel wrapped up tight. In Mothercare I treated myself to a couple of tops, a nightie and pair of pyjamas. They were all suitable for breastfeeding with discreet little openings and I cracked Dave up with a demo of them all later - they would be more appropriate at an Ann Summers party!

Thursday 22nd May

We went for another appointment with the midwife in the morning. Ruth said my blood test results and measurements were all good but when she felt for Pear she said she thought he may be in the breech position. I had only just been reading about breech babies in one of my pregnancy books as I couldn't work out which way up he was from the strange assortment of hands and feet he kept sticking out. She did say not to worry as most breech babies drop to the correct position between 32 and 36 weeks.

Dave and I went back to 'Lili May' to order a crib for Pear that should be in stock in two weeks. We had chosen a lovely white oval shaped one, that started off quite small and then as your baby grew there were extra pieces you could add to increase the size. It should last him until he is 7 years old and then the crib can be split in half to make 2 cool chairs.

Later on I got a bit tearful - even though the midwife said not to be too concerned at this point about Pear being breech I couldn't help but worry, it's what I do best! I read everything in my pregnancy book about helping to turn your baby to a better position for birth and one thing that appealed to me the most was Hypnotherapy - most likely because it is totally non-invasive. The statistics of it helping were extremely good and so I went online to do a bit more research. I came across an amazing site all about HypnoBirthing that sounded brilliant. In short, it explained that by taking classes you could learn to relax and free yourself from any fears and in doing so prevent the fear-tension-pain syndrome. As well as helping correct breech presentations other benefits included - less likelihood of medical intervention and painkillers, a reduced first stage of labour, less pelvic floor damage, a more speedy recovery from the birth, increased bonding with your baby and a peaceful and natural birth, with a calm and alert baby. It emphasized the links between your mind, your body and your baby all working together in harmony to enable a beautiful birthing, free from pain.

I was sold on all of the points I read, HypnoBirthing classes sounded perfect for me especially with my fear of all things medical. I showed Dave my findings and he agreed, so I wrote down the details and planned to give the lady a call the next day to find out when her next classes were and if she had any availabilities.

Friday 23rd May

I had a few aches and pains last night - hunger pains I think from staying up so late on the computer.

Our bathroom was delivered today but disappointingly quite a few items were damaged so we had to go into the store to get them replaced.

When we got back in I found time to ring up about the HypnoBirthing classes. I spoke to a lovely lady called Karen Knight whose company was delightfully named 'Hypnobabes'. I instantly hit it off with her and she patiently answered lots of questions I had about the content of the classes. It turned out she was part way through a course but as we had only missed one session we could have a private class with her on Monday and then join the rest of her class on Tuesday night. I was buzzing with excitement when I got off the phone, I had wanted to sort out antenatal classes for a while and this has just fallen into place perfectly.

Sunday 25th May

Poor Dave had a bit of an accident today when he was trying to take out the old toilet cistern - the ceramic cracked and sliced a big chunk off his thumb! He calmly came upstairs asking for a plaster, I had my back to him and when I looked around there was blood pouring everywhere! Amazingly - for me - I stayed incredibly calm and did my best first aid bandage ever, as well as getting him to elevate his arm to stop the bleeding.

I was finding it difficult to walk past 'JoJo Maman Bébé' without being tempted to go inside and peruse all their lovely mum and baby products and once again I found myself drawn in. I had been using a product called 'Mama Mio Tummy Rub Stretch Mark Oil' and absolutely loved it. In the store I noticed that they had the entire 'Mama Mio' range including a 'Tummy Rub Stretch Mark Butter' to rub in on top of the oil as your tummy increased in size. There was also some lotion called 'Boob Tube', which promised to nourish and protect this delicate area as well as helping to keep your boobs firm - fingers crossed! I treated myself to both and got my loyalty card stamped; at this rate I would soon have a full card and when I did I would get £15 off my next purchase.

After dinner we went for a walk up the seafront to see a firework display but it was so windy and Pear was kicking me lots so we left early.

Monday 26th May

I spent the day doing bits and pieces around the house and flitted between looking forward to our HypnoBirthing class in the evening and worrying it might be too hypnotizing for me! I needn't have worried as Karen and her partner Jason put us totally at our ease and we learnt so much in the 4 hours we were there. A lot of what Karen talked about was along a similar vein to a brilliant book I had been reading recently called 'A Spiritual Midwife' by Ina May Gaskin. We watched a couple of DVDs of women giving birth without pain-relief and experiencing no pain - I wanted that! We finished our session and came away with a HypnoBirthing book and folder to collect all the coursework we would be receiving in. I was so glad we decided to enrol in this class; I thought it would be great for both of us. As well as helping me to overcome any fears I might have, HypnoBirthing classes placed a strong focus on the importance of your partner and were aimed at helping him to become confident, supportive and protective like a silverback gorilla.

Tuesday 27th May

Dave got his thumb checked out by a nurse today and she complimented me on my bandaging skills - I did get my first aid badge in Brownies!

In the evening we went to our 2nd HypnoBirthing class and met the other two couples who were absolutely lovely. The evening whizzed by - we learnt how to do a light finger massage, did some very relaxing guided hypnosis and watched a DVD of a woman having a water birth with no drama or pain. Karen gave us a 'Rainbow Relaxation' CD to listen to every night in bed which we did as soon as we got home.

Tips and things to do

- All five of your baby's senses are functional now and he or she weighs around 4 pounds.

- Your uterus will be pushing all your organs everyway but don't worry they will eventually make their way back after the birth! As you get larger eating and sleeping becomes more difficult. I continued snacking at night and started sleeping with a couple of pillows propping me up as well as one under my knees which seemed to help.

- Relax as much as possible and try to refrain from going too crazy starting any large projects that you may not finish in time.

- Keep drinking plenty of water and make sure you get enough fibre in your diet - I had organic bran flakes in my yoghurt every morning.

- You may need to get yet another bra fitted around now - yes I know your boobs have a mind of their own! It's really important to have a supportive, comfy bra.

- Starting an antenatal class is a great way to prepare yourself for the birth of your baby. It is great if you can attend one with your partner as he will feel much more part of the experience. There are several different kinds for you to choose from, some may be free of charge and others may cost varying amounts. The NCT offer classes and there may be private companies in your area offering Active Birth classes or HypnoBirthing classes like the one we attended. Have a search on-line; ask friends for recommendations and select a course you both feel will be the most beneficial to you. Depending on the type of class you choose you may find they focus on different things. What is important to you? Do you want to concentrate on just the birth, learn about parenting, relaxation techniques and exercises to help before and after the birth, or join a group to make friends with other couples in the same situation? We found that the course we chose ticked all the boxes and hopefully you will find a class to suit your needs too.

WEEK 33

The ****it bucket...

Wednesday 28th May

There was no yoga today as it was half term so instead I met up with my new friend Cheryl, from class. I most definitely had my pregnancy brain switched on as I waited for her in the wrong coffee shop, but fortunately we tracked each other down - eventually. I gave her a pink change bag as she knew she was having a little girl and she gave me a cute blue bodysuit for Pear. It was great having a girly chat and comparing notes about our bumps, ailments, etc.

I had another nice chat in the evening on the phone to my mum, I told her all about our HypnoBirthing classes and she agreed that they sounded great. Mum was on a mission to try and guess our baby's name - despite me telling her that we were keeping it a secret. She was desperate to have a go at guessing and had me in hysterics. Our conversation went a bit like this -

Mum: '*You know you have been calling him Pear, well, I think you are going to keep that name but spell it Pier as in Brighton Pier!*'

Me: 'No *mum it's not that, we haven't tried to be clever choosing a name it's just one we both like*'.

Mum: '*I've got it where did you go on your honeymoon?*'

Me: '*We are not calling him Orlando!*'

Mum: '*No think about it, where in Orlando did you go? Disneyland...*'

Me: '*I give up, you're being too lateral*'.

Mum: '*Mickey as in Mickey Mouse!*'

Thursday 29th May

The day started off really sunny so Dave made the most of it and cleared out our old car as it was getting sold on Saturday to a guy off ebay.

I busied myself doing housewifey things - changing the sheets, putting the laundry on and even made fresh pizza for lunch.

Things went a bit downhill when the phone rang and it was our tenant in Folkestone saying that the ceiling had water leaking through it, again! I rang the managing agents to let them know and had a bit of a moan, but as always it fell on deaf ears and all I succeeded in doing was winding myself up. I got off the phone and had a bit of a cry and Pear flipped around in sympathy or distress too. I decided to take some advice that Karen, our HypnoBirthing teacher, had given us in the last lesson we did. She said if something was stressing you out and you felt as though you had no control over the situation then to imagine you had what she described as a '****it bucket' and to put whatever was bothering you in it. I tried it out and did actually feel a bit better, after all there wasn't anything physically that I could do so there was no point getting wound up about it.

Later on in the day it started to rain but we ventured out for some fresh air and discovered another wonderful baby shop nearby called 'Yummies' that was an Aladdin's Cave of baby clothes, toys and trinkets. I bought Pear a gorgeous vest bodysuit by 'Green Baby' with lots of blue pears on it, one of which had a little bite taken out of it - very cute.

Friday 30th May
The bits and pieces we ordered for the bathroom that had been damaged got re-delivered today so we could get started on the bathroom soon.

Nick and Catherine came to see us and were so complimentary about all the things we had done to the place since they were last here. It was a real moral boost as sometimes it felt as if we were making hardly any progress at all.

They took us out to The George for a lovely lunch; it was so warm we sat outside in the beer garden. Afterwards we went for a wander to the beach and then stopped at Dave's favourite ice cream parlour where once again they treated us. I had a delicious vegan rhubarb and blackberry sorbet that was totally yummy. It was such a lovely day spent with lovely people. By the evening I was absolutely exhausted from all the walking and talking!

Saturday 31st May
I had a great night's sleep, I think our social day yesterday wore Pear out too as he didn't keep me awake

kicking as usual. I even managed to make a few trips to the toilet without doing myself a mishap on the bath that was propped up in the hallway.

Dave started filling some big holes we had in our bedroom windows, as when it was windy he could feel it blowing in and it gave him a stiff neck.

I went up the high street to transfer some money into our joint account as our London tenants were late paying their rent which might put us over our over-draft limit. I also picked up the ingredients to make a vegan baked cheesecake I had a craving for. It was incredibly busy everywhere and very hot so I headed home and spent the afternoon baking and preparing a roast for dinner. In the evening 4 guys came to pick up the car, which was a bit disconcerting at first but they seemed nice enough and the one who was buying it said he was getting it for his dad. We exchanged the keys for his cash and he headed off happy with his purchase. Even though we were sad to see the car go, we were glad of the money he gave us for it.

Sunday 1st June

I didn't sleep very well last night as little Pear was squirming around for ages. I wanted to sleep on my side but didn't as I was worried I would squash his arm or leg or whatever it was he kept sticking out. I did eventually get a couple of hours sleep and then made up for it by laying in until 11 am - I had to make the most of lie-ins as I knew when Pear arrived they would become a thing of the past.

I spoke to my dad on the phone later and ordered some books online for him for Father's Day.

Dave made a start on the bathroom by painting the ceiling - hooray! We decided that although the ceiling was pretty ancient and would be best taken down and re-plastered, we simply didn't have the time to get it done before Pear made his entrance (well not if we hoped to have a fully functioning bathroom that was). We were a bit worried that painting the ceiling might result in the old plaster coming away but it looked fine - double hooray!

While the paint dried Dave and I took a walk down to the beach - I didn't think I could ever tire of looking at the sea, it was so calming and beautiful.

In the evening I cooked dinner and watched some TV while Dave painted the bathroom walls - gone was the cool blue replaced with a much warmer shade of cream, the same as the bedroom and hallway.

Monday 2nd June

I stayed in during the day, happy just pottering around while Dave carried on with the bathroom. I was chief tea and food maker which meant he was getting more done as he didn't keep stopping to make his own - what a hard taskmaster I was!

In the evening we drove to our HypnoBirthing class and had an enjoyable session again - the classes had become the highlight of our week. With all the D.I.Y. going on at home it was great to go out and have a chance to reconnect with each other in such a relaxing environment. Karen made everyone feel so at home and knew how to keep Dave happy with delicious coconut and chocolate biscuits on hand. Tonight we learnt how to release fears - Karen led us through guided self-hypnosis where we imagined being in a hot air balloon with a box containing any fears we might have beside us. One by one we visualised throwing them out of the balloon and them falling over a stretch of water where they eventually sunk and vanished. Afterwards we all felt really relaxed, so I would definitely be practicing that one out at home as I had lots of fears to try it out on! We were also given some ideas for our birth plan which was great as we should probably write one soon in case Pear decided to arrive early. When we got home I had a bath and then Dave and I snuggled up in bed to read our HypnoBirthing book. We had been taking it in turns to read and were really enjoying doing it together. Our usual evening routine would consist of us zoned out watching TV and occasionally grunting at each other so reading aloud was a major improvement! We fell asleep listening to our 'Rainbow Relaxation' CD - zzzzzzzzzzzzzzz.

Tuesday 3rd June

I listened to my 'Affirmations for an easy birth' CD when I woke up. It was lovely with soft music playing in the background and lots of positive affirmations such as - I put all fear aside as I prepare for the birth of my baby, I am relaxed and happy that my baby is finally coming to me, I am focused on a smooth, easy birth, I trust my body to know what to do, I feel confident, safe and secure. My favourite affirmation was - I welcome my baby with happiness and joy.

Dave and I were booked in for a free antenatal class at our midwife centre in the morning. Part of me was keen to go and meet other mums-to-be and part of me was apprehensive and a bit worried that there might be negativity and scare stories that would undo the good from our HypnoBirthing classes.

As it turned out everyone was lovely, especially the couple sat next to us. We exchanged numbers with them so we could hopefully stay in touch. The midwife running the course was friendly and jolly, she covered all the basics without adding any unnecessary gore! There was one woman in the group - the mother of a pregnant lady - who just couldn't stop regaling everyone with all her horror stories from the numerous babies she had given birth to. Dave and I kept looking at each other and smiling, while at the same time trying to ignore what she was saying I just imagined my hands over my ears and saying la la la! Thankfully after a couple of attempts to scare every pregnant woman in the room the midwife cut her short and steered the conversation back to more pleasant and useful topics. When she put a DVD on of a tour of the local hospital I decided to pop to the loo in case it showed any scary caesareans or ventouse births. I had a bit of a theory of my own about all the information and films shown to pregnant women, at a time in your life when you were at your most vulnerable. I personally really disliked going to the dentist - was almost phobic about it. Now if I needed a root canal treatment I knew for a fact that it would not make me feel any more confident if the dentist asked me if I would like to watch a film of someone else having one done - no thank you!

When I returned to the room I caught the end of the hospital tour, which they now show on TV rather than letting couples visit, to prevent the spread of germs. Dave and I had already decided that if we had the choice we would like to have Pear at home. I knew some people felt more confident surrounded by machinery and technology but it frightened the life out of me. I must have got my dislike of hospitals from when I was 2 years old and had a big operation - I still remember the lights above the operating table. Even now if I go to visit someone else in hospital I have this fear that a man in a white coat is going to take me away - probably not a bad idea! So for us home would be best, with all my creature comforts around me.

After the session another lady came in to discuss breastfeeding with us - we had all been asked to bring a doll or teddy bear in for this part. Dave and I got the giggles when we looked around at everyone else's 'babies' that were all new and appropriately dressed. I had brought my teddy from birth with me, Queenie. She was actually a Sooty bear but she had a bit of a sex change when I renamed her and also promoted her to queen of all my toys. Over the years she had been fed Marmite, drank Ribena and her paws had been re-stitched numerous times. One look at her and you could see she had been well loved and in this group she was causing a few smiles especially as she had no clothes on! I wrapped her up in the blanket we had also been asked to bring along and tried not to make eye contact with Dave - who was struggling to come to grips with watching a roomful of women attempting to breastfeed an assortment of soft toys - surreal to say the least! It all seemed straightforward enough if a little unreal doing it on something that didn't mind being dangled upside down while you switched sides.

After the class Dave and I went to the tip with yet more rubbish - we were here so often I wouldn't be surprised if they gave us our own skip with a little plaque on it.

We did a big shop at Sainsbury's and were going to go to Tesco afterwards for some veggie burgers, but both of us were so exhausted by then that we decided to go home and 'veg' out ourselves instead.

Tips and things to do

- Your baby is gaining fat which turns the skin from red to a pinker colour. He or she now measures about 43 cm or 17 inches from top to toe.

- You will be gaining about a pound a week around now, continue to eat well and get lots of rest.

- Have you started thinking about baby names yet? Before we knew Pear was going to be a boy I tried out several names both male and female on him. When I lay in the bath I would ask him to kick me if he liked them - one kick for yes two for no! We only ever had one boys name that stood out for us and that was Cole. I used to watch a TV show called 'Charmed' about three sisters who were witches, had magical powers and fought evil. One of the main male characters was called Cole - he was half human, half demon but to his defence his human half was gorgeous, even if during a few episodes he did become the source of all things evil! I loved the name and it also helped that the actor playing Cole was the dishy Julian McMahon of 'Nip Tuck' fame and I can see quite a few similarities between him and my hubby. The only thing we struggled with was coming up with a second name for Cole. I wanted something that began with a J so that Cole would have the choice to be CJ if he wanted. The names we came up with were Jaxon and Jayden and with our tried and tested kick-o-meter Jayden it was!

- When you are choosing a name for your baby a good piece of advice I read was to choose a name that would suit a poet, lawyer or rock star and always choose something both you and your partner are happy with, don't feel obliged to name your baby after some long lost Aunt or Uncle twice removed! I spent many a happy hour at the shops browsing through books that gave the meanings to names.

- Avoid getting caught up in other people's birth stories especially if they are negative tales that will stick in your head and maybe effect your own baby's birth. Karen, our HypnoBirth teacher, suggested we ask the question, 'Is what you're about to tell me, going to help me have a calm and relaxed birth?' That prevented any horror stories from being relayed to us!

The week I burst my birth ball!

Wednesday 4th June

I had an enjoyable yoga class in the morning; Dom had us all very relaxed at the end of the session as she talked us through a lovely visualisation where we imagined we were breathing in the sea air.

When I got home Dave was just finishing off painting in the bathroom so we decided to make the most of the sunshine and got some real sea air.

We sat on the beach, Dave with his legs in a mini box split and I sat between them leaning back against his chest. It was a very comfy position for me, not so much for Dave. I read some more of our HypnoBirthing book out loud and we chatted to Pear. It was such a lovely way to pass the afternoon - sunshine, sea and wonderful company, what more could I ask for? As we walked back home I felt out of breath and my tummy felt really weird, kind of stretched and very hard. I wondered if it was a 'Braxton Hicks' contraction that I had been reading about, but the sensation was quite different to how they were described. Maybe like lots of things in pregnancy it varied between women.

By the time we got home the weirdness had passed thankfully, as it wasn't a particularly pleasant feeling. The post had been delivered and Pear's 'Symphony in Motion' crib mobile had arrived. We got it out the box and had a little play around with it. It consisted of a music box you attached to the crib that played Mozart, Beethoven and Bach while the mobile moved overhead with its black and white swirly patterns and zoo animals in bright colours. We packed away the mobile part but kept out the music box to play to Pear so that he became familiar with it. We were both pretty impressed with the quality of the music as it actually was recognisable as classical music and not at all 'plinky-plonky', as Dave described some of the other mobiles we had heard. After all we were going to be hearing quite a bit of it over the next few months - as would our tenant downstairs, so it needed to be bearable.

Thursday 5th June

I had a really up and down sort of a day today. It started off well with our mortgage offer finally coming through which was a relief financially - or at least would be when we got the money in our bank account.

I found myself getting a bit overwhelmed and tearful at the quantity of things that still needed doing in the bathroom before it was fully functional. Having to fill a bucket every time you used the loo to flush it was wearing thin. Dave rang his brother John to see if he would be up for coming over for a couple of days to help us and he said yes...Yay!

Our lovely tenant from downstairs popped by to hand in her notice as she was moving back to Guernsey which was such a shame as she had been great. It also meant that rather than running her tenancy on we would most likely end up having to repaint and clean a few bits and pieces downstairs - at a time when to be honest we had more than enough on our own plates...typical.

I rang all our mortgage companies in the afternoon to see if we were eligible to take a mortgage break or payment holiday. One of them said yes there and then on the phone that we could have 3 months break and another one said that if I sent in a 'Mat B1 form' that proved I was pregnant that we could have 6 months break from 2 of our mortgages. I felt like having a little cartwheel when I got off the phone, but refrained.

In the evening my gum suddenly started bleeding and on closer inspection it looked like I had a blister near where my new inlay was. It eventually stopped and I swished my mouth with some of Dave's antibacterial mouthwash and kept my fingers crossed that it would sort itself out as I didn't want to be paying the dentist another visit so soon. What a funny old day.

Friday 6th June

I slept well last night and woke feeling refreshed and full of beans. After a fresh fruit smoothie for breakfast Dave and I wandered up to the health centre to pick up a 'Mat B1 form' for our mortgage company. It was another beautiful day that made us feel so glad to be enjoying it and not grinding away at work. The receptionist at the centre explained that they didn't have a form to hand but that we could pop back later to pick one up.

I made a start on tidying up our small garden area at the front of our flat, as there was a bush that had totally taken over the entire bed. I trimmed it back and pinched some earth for a couple of indoor pot plants we had, that were only just surviving on the tiniest bit of dry old earth.

Later we picked up the form and got it off in the post to the mortgage company so it was quite a productive day all in all.

Sunday 8th June

There was a Baby Expo on at the Brighton Centre today so Dave and I tootled down to check it out. It seemed as though the rest of Brighton had the same idea. I had never seen so many pregnant women and pushchairs in one area - it was quite overwhelming. We chatted to an independent midwife and also a lovely doula, both of whom were aware of the HypnoBirthing course we were participating in and were very positive and open to it. At the moment I was leaning towards having a doula as everything I had read about them had sounded really good. Their role if you like was to mother the mother, which in the society we live in where many mums and daughters live so far away from each other - my mum is some 4 hours drive away - was a comforting thought. They are there to act as a go between, passing your wishes on to the midwives and supporting you and your partner. Statistics say that couples choosing to use the services of a doula are less likely to need medical intervention - a big plus in my books. The doula we chatted to was called Samsara Tanner and we instantly hit it off with her. As a mother of 4 children herself she was a joy to talk to and a real 'Earth Mother' who clearly saw her job not as work but as a blessing which was refreshing. We took her details and decided to have a little think about it at home later.

There was a stand with 'Mother-ease' reusable nappies that I had been reading about on the internet.

I was particularly taken with their range made from bamboo as they felt incredibly soft which if I were a baby I would choose for comfort. The company was having a special offer on purchases made on the day but we were going to hold on until we were 100 percent sure they were the ones we wanted to get.

A trip to the toilet resulted in me picking up lots of free samples - kindly left in there - of different brands and sizes of bio-disposable nappies. They would come in handy the first few days and could go in my birth bag.

We took a break from the hustle and bustle of the exhibition centre to sit on the beach with a sandwich and cold drink, mmmmmh!

When we got home Dave carried on with the laminate flooring in the hallway, that was only half finished and I made a scrummy vegan cheesecake for pudding later.

John arrived in the afternoon; I made us all a roast dinner and we devoured most of the cheesecake. Dave's mum rang in the evening and we all took it in turns chatting to her. In bed later I got a bit of a stomach ache and when my customary yoghurt didn't do the trick Dave put on our 'Rainbow Relaxation' CD and I fell asleep straight away which was brilliant.

Monday 9th June

What a day!

Today Dave had big plans of making an early start of the huge list of D.I.Y. we still had to do. Unfortunately after all his driving yesterday John didn't wake up very early and it was nearly 12 pm before they were ready to make a start on things. Dave was stuck in to the bathroom and didn't really need help so I decided to ask John to go into the dreaded loft to retrieve some more of my treasures. Bless him it was such a hot day and the loft was probably another 10 degrees hotter so it wasn't a fun job. I stood at the bottom of the ladder trying to remember what exactly it was I wanted passing down, whilst avoiding the odd item of clothing that would fall down every now and then. After a while we were both feeling decidedly hot and flustered; John desperate to come down and me itching to get up there myself. In the end I rather foolishly decided to pull my birth ball into the doorway to supervise from there. Big mistake - huge! I must have dragged it past a screw that was sticking out of the side of a small shelving unit John had passed down. One minute I was gently bouncing, the next there was this enormous bang and I was on my back with my legs in the air and the shelf had fallen on top of me!

Unbelievably John didn't notice and carried on sorting through things overhead, while Dave bombed up the stairs to see me under a pile of stuff on the floor still trying to work out if I was about to give birth!

He got me downstairs to the bedroom, I couldn't stop shaking I was so shocked - I am rubbish if anyone pops a balloon at a party and this sounded like a gun going off. Amazingly Pear seemed to rather enjoy the whole experience and started jumping up and down. (I hoped he was not going to grow up an adrenaline junkie with me at home worrying myself silly about what he was up to). I thought my waters might have broken during the fall but was mortified and also rather relieved to discover it was wee! - Note to self: I should have done more pelvic floor exercises. I telephoned the maternity unit and explained what had happened and when the midwife had stopped giggling she assured me I should be fine and that babies are resilient little things.

We had an uneventful afternoon and Pear did eventually calm down after his bungee jump!

In the evening Dave and I drove to our HypnoBirthing class - they were all quite amused by my birth ball mishap and now I knew why the ball was so cheap, as it didn't have a double layer that would have protected against bursting. Our class was lovely - as well as being informative about what to expect during the birth we learnt some breathing exercises, watched some more DVDs of women having natural, easy births and did some relaxation exercises and self-hypnosis.

Tuesday 10th June

I slept so well last night. I still hadn't managed to stay awake through the entire 'Rainbow Relaxation' CD.

Dave and John went to Tesco and took some rubbish to the tip while I washed my hair, tidied the kitchen and took some ID to our financial advisor as she couldn't find a record of me on her system.

After lunch John made a start on painting our stairwell and landing for us. I felt so useless and frustrated as painting was usually my thing, although there was no way I could have hung over the stairs - pregnant or not.

Tips and things to do

- If you do buy a birth ball don't make the mistake we did and scrimp on it as you most definitely need an anti-burst ball.

- See if there are any baby shows in your area. They are great places for picking up tips and advice. You may also get to meet local independent midwives and doulas in your area as well as picking up some useful freebies.

- Start thinking where you would like to have your baby - home, hospital or maybe a birthing unit. Don't let other people influence your choice and try to put you off whatever decision you have made. As I mentioned previously I have a bit of a fear of hospitals so Dave and I decided we would try for a home birth and if any special circumstances arose we could always transfer to hospital. Below is my list of pros and cons of hospital and home birth.

Hospital
Scared of hospitals
Worried about mistakes such as being given the wrong baby!
Maybe dirty
Dave may not be able to stay with me over night
Rubbish food - unlikely to have any vegan choices
Good if something should go wrong

Home birth
Will feel more relaxed being in familiar surroundings
Less likely to have medical intervention
Get the same midwife, maybe even two
Dave can stay with me the entire time
I can use the bath/birth pool
Can eat what I like, when I like
Can still transfer to hospital if I need to

- Your baby is starting to develop immunities to help fight mild infections.

- You may find you experience more 'Braxton Hicks' contractions.

- If you are working you may decide to start your Maternity leave soon. Some women like to work for as long as possible and so have more leave time with their baby. It's a personal choice and you could find you change your mind - several times - as to when to take it from.

- Keep drinking plenty of water to combat swollen ankles.

- You could maybe spend a day having a cook-up of all your favourite meals to freeze.

- Spend an evening with your partner having a look at your finances together. There are maybe still a few big items you need to purchase so try to budget for them. Talk about how you plan to manage financially when your baby arrives, do you need to look into childcare etc?

- Write your birth preferences down, this is known as a birth plan. I like the idea of it being called birth preferences as that implies you have choices and can change to account for the situation.

Here is ours:

We are planning a Homebirth using HypnoBirthing, which is based on having a birth as natural and relaxing as possible using breathing and relaxation techniques. We therefore kindly request your help with the following:

We plan to use breathing, relaxation and self-hypnosis techniques and the use of a water birthing pool to keep the birth as natural and drug free as possible.

We would really appreciate if you could support us in our techniques that require peace and quiet. If you could avoid using any references to 'pain', 'hurt', 'hard labour' or any suggestion of pain being experienced. We would also prefer the word 'contraction' to be substituted with 'surge' also for 'pushing' to be replaced with 'breathing or nudging down the baby'.

I do not want an induced labour unless necessary for medical reasons, with time for discussion.

We would like to use natural stimulation in the event of a stalled or slow labour.

During labour I would like to remain free to move about as much as possible to find the most comfortable positions.

I would like monitoring to occur only if necessary and minimal vaginal exams - and only with permission.

For delivery whatever position feels most comfortable.

For our baby to be delivered straight to my tummy for skin to skin contact.

For you to help me breastfeed correctly.

I would request that the placenta delivery to occur naturally without the aid of an injection.

To delay the cutting of the cord until it has finished pulsating.

For our baby please allow the vernix to be absorbed into his skin. Please could you delay 'cleaning or rubbing' and use a soft cloth when rubbing is appropriate.

Orgasmic birth!

Wednesday 11th June

I got a bit upset in my yoga class today when Dom asked us to lie on our right side and I just couldn't. Pear wasn't having any of it and it felt as though I had a hamster running backwards round a wheel in my tummy. I was getting myself a bit worked up that he might be in the wrong position as whenever I looked at my HypnoBirthing pictures of the optimal position for birthing I couldn't figure out where Pear was exactly but it felt as though he was on the diagonal instead of his head being directly down. My pregnancy book reassured me that there still was time for him to drop into the correct position so I would just have to stay focused and positive, as it was pointless worrying myself silly about something that might or might not be the case anyway.

After class Cheryl and I went to The Pavilion for a catch up - she was starting a HypnoBirthing class with Karen tonight so that was cool as we would be able to compare notes.

When I got home Dave was still hard at it in the bathroom and John was finishing up painting the stairway.

Reinforcements arrived in the afternoon in the shape of Janet and Tony who had also taken pity on our predicament and kindly offered their services. They had some refreshments with us and a chat, then left to find their campsite as they were staying in their campervan.

Thursday 12th June

It was a bit of a hectic day today; Dave and John went to the tip to dump yet more debris from the bathroom and John's car broke down. While John waited for the RAC, Dave and I nipped out as I had to see the midwife. After my usual pee on a stick routine she informed me that I had a bit of protein in my urine, but didn't seem unduly worried saying it might just be because I hadn't drunk much so far today. Great news Pear was in the right position...Yay! I spent the rest of the afternoon telling him how clever he was and hoping he didn't flip around - maybe my accident on the birth ball did the trick.

Janet and Tony came over and we caught up over a cuppa and some cake, we didn't get much done as in the evening Dave and I went to see a film at The Meeting House with the catchy name 'Orgasmic Birth'! We met Karen and the other couples from our HypnoBirthing class there and sat together. Thankfully we weren't in the front row as the first bit of the film was rather graphic - or so I assumed - as I scooted down on my chair behind the person in front of me so I couldn't actually see the ventouse birth being performed. Karen nudged me when it was safe to watch again and the rest of the film was as the title suggested 'orgasmic'. Amazingly there were women all experiencing natural - and from the expressions on their faces really enjoyable - births. One lady giving birth in a gorgeous outdoor pool with lots of little candles dotted around was having such a good time her eyes crossed in ecstasy. By the end of the film we all came away saying we would like some of that, how brilliant would it be to have no pain just pure pleasure - we would have to wait and see how it panned out for us.

Friday 13th June

I was having a lovely sleep until 4 am when the next door neighbours decided to hold an impromptu party judging from the loud music. I eventually dozed off and got up at the deliciously decadent time of 10 am.

Janet and Tony came around at 11 am and made a start on sanding down the window sills in the living room and banisters in the hallway. Strangely I felt a bit tearful, hormonal and stressed out with everyone. After practically begging Dave to get us some help I was finding it hard to relinquish control and let my lovely team of helpers get on with it. It didn't sit comfortably with me watching everyone else beavering away while I did nothing apart from make a steady supply of tea and coffee. In the end I dragged my useless self out the house for a walk up the high street to put our remortgage cheque in the bank. Seeing our bank account looking healthy for the first time in ages really lifted my spirits and I nipped in M&S for doughnuts for the workforce.

Saturday 14th June

Painting was about to commence at last today until we made the discovery that we had run out of paint and a trip to the vegan paint shop was fruitless as unbelievably they didn't have any left either...growl!

Instead we all went for a nice lunch at Kensington's and tummies full - mine particularly so - we got stuck into the flat on our return. Janet found a tin of paint with a few dregs in it that she managed to stretch quite a way over the banisters and Tony filled some massive holes in the window sills and did yet more sanding, bless him.

I had another bash at the bush outside, determined to pull it up as I had big plans to deck this little area out the front so Pear would have some outdoor space, albeit miniscule.

Sunday 15th June

Janet and Tony had a well deserved day off today to explore the surrounding area. Dave was up to the stage of taking our toilet out completely so they had chosen wisely. I felt pretty tired, so I spent a few hours reading in the library where at least I knew there was a functioning toilet. I treated Dave to a veggie burger from 'Red Veg' and kept him company as he worked for a couple of hours, until I needed the loo so I headed off to a book-store for a wee and yet more reading. I stayed there until 5 pm, when they booted us all out and I was really pleased to see Dave had made major progress in our bathroom. He had the laminate flooring down and half the toilet in, so even if nothing more got done we were in the same position as before in that we could use the loo and flush it by pouring a bucket of water down the pan.

We had such a relaxing evening together, Dave read the rest of our HypnoBirthing book to me which was great.

Monday 16th June

Dave managed to get our paint today and we left Janet and Tony to it while we went to the tip and Tesco's. We bought an obscene amount of food - stock piling in case

Pear got wind of the fact we had nearly finished the bathroom and arrived early!

I bought some beautiful lilies for Karen as tonight was sadly our last HypnoBirthing class. It was a lovely long session the best part of 4 hours. Dave and I both felt so much more prepared and confident for doing the course, but we would miss the classes; Monday nights just wouldn't be the same.

Tuesday 17th June

Janet and Tony headed home today - they had done such a great job with the painting and we were both so grateful to them. The flat felt really empty and quiet with just the two of us again. The absolute highlight of the day/month was when Dave finally got the new toilet working. Now I never thought I would get excited about something as utilitarian as a loo, but then the never ending buckets of water had been a pain to say the least. This one was fantastic - the 'Rolls Royce' of loos - complete with a slow closing seat you could just let go of...cool.

I must have been sitting in the same position for too long last night as my back started really hurting. It was such a lovely sunny day so we wandered/hobbled to the bank but I had to keep stopping as my back was aching so much. When we got home I found a bit of relief by lying on a pile of pillows on the living room floor, I hoped it would only be temporary as I didn't want to be suffering with a dodgy back for the rest of my pregnancy.

Tips and things to do

- This week the average baby weighs about 5½ pounds and fills most of your uterus so you may not feel him or her moving around as much.

- From now on every time you visit your midwife she will check the position of your baby. Try not to worry too much even if your baby isn't in the optimal position, there is still plenty of time and most babies do drop to a good position. You could put pictures around the house showing the best position - I had one near my bed, in the bathroom and even on the fridge! Each time you look at the picture imagine your baby in that position and gently talk to him or her about it.

- As your tummy grows reaching your toenails to clip them becomes almost impossible, treat yourself to a pedicure.

- Take time each day to relax with your feet up and a good book. I kept re-reading all my favourite pregnancy books especially the ones that listed things that were happening on a weekly basis to me and my baby.

- Even though you may not feel like it, try to keep up some gentle exercise such as walking and swimming. I didn't find out until after I had my baby that just a couple of streets away from us there was a special mum and baby pool called 'Little Dippers'. As well as the water being a lovely warm temperature it offered special relaxation sessions for pregnant ladies. I know with my love of the bath if I had been aware of its existence sooner I would have been there every night!

- A little reminder for you - pelvic floor and squats. You will be so glad you did them, trust me.

- Decide if you would like to have a baby shower. I would have loved one but as my friends were all miles away it didn't seem very practical. If you do fancy having one drop hints to your best friend, I'm sure she would enjoy organising one for you.

- If you are a big softy like me you could write a letter to your baby to put in their keepsake box for when they are older. Here is mine:

Dearest darling baby Pear,

We just wanted to let you know how much we are looking forward to meeting you at your birth day.

You have been planned for, wanted and anticipated for so long now and your existence is our very own little miracle.

As you grow in my tummy I already feel I know you. Your personality is already showing through. You are considerate, sensitive and very clever. When I need reassurance that you are OK you always respond with a kick or a wiggle which never fails to delight us.

Your daddy and I cherish the time we spend bonding with you. Not a day goes past without us talking to you, including you in all our plans for our future together. We especially love singing to you in the bath. You most definitely recognise your songs and our voices.

As my body changes and my bump grows in size, I feel so proud. You are amazing and I am doing everything I can to eat well, to nurture you. You already can taste what I am eating and have shown a liking for fresh fruit smoothies, yoghurt and dark chocolate and even just a couple of pieces set you dancing around - just like your daddy!

As your birth day gets closer your daddy and I are trying to get our home ready for you. We would love for you to be born here in safe and familiar surroundings. We are working hard at our classes to give us all a stress and pain free birth. We dream of you arriving in the world here at home surrounded by love, with dim lighting, candles, soft music and relaxing aromatherapy oils. We trust that you will get yourself into the best position for birth and that together with my body you will have an easy, relaxing birth.

We imagine holding you in our arms and introducing you to the world. All your grandparents, aunts and uncles are really looking forward to meeting you and showering you with lots of love and affection.

If we could give you a blessing it would be that all your life you have fantastic health, great happiness and good fortune.

We promise to love you and to teach you everything we know, with patience and kindness and also to learn from you. Know that as you grow we will always be here for you to love and support you.

All our love

Your mummy and daddy xx

Homebirth meeting...

Wednesday 18th June

No Cheryl at yoga today so I hoped she was OK. My back felt a lot better so that was a relief. Dave was still working on the bathroom when I got home so I busied myself tidying the living room as it was very dusty from all the sanding.

Karen emailed me that there was a homebirth meeting at a local couple's home later so Dave and I decided to go along. It was a really good evening; there were about 8 other couples there as well, so we were all squeezed into their sitting room. The main thing that we and most of the other couples wanted to know was; what to do if when we telephoned the hospital saying we required a midwife for a homebirth that they tried to get us to change our minds and come into hospital instead. We were told that - at the sake of sounding like a broken record - to keep just repeating, 'We are having a homebirth and require a midwife'. Apparently it was best if the mum-to-be didn't speak on the phone as she was more likely to get talked into changing her plans. Ideally a friend, or if you employed the services of a doula they could do the honours as they were more likely to remain steadfast in relaying your wishes. By the end of the evening we felt a lot more confident about having a homebirth. I had been getting a bit concerned that we may end up really disappointed, if after making the huge decision to have Pear at home, that for no other reason than logistics we were not able to.

Thursday 19th June

We made an effort to get up early as we had so many things to do. Top of the list was getting rid of yet more stuff at the tip; a car full again!

After the tip we went to B&Q and Wickes to look at tiles for the bathroom and kitchen. I quite fancied some plain rectangular ones that I thought would compliment the bath and units we had already. In Wickes we found some inexpensive white ones and also got some exactly the same in black for the kitchen.

By the time we got home it was 6 pm and I was so tired plus Pear was sticking his 'little tools' out all night. Dave and I joked that he had a Black& Decker sander in there with him.

Friday 20th June

Dave got started with the tiling in the bathroom and I was very pleased with our choice as they looked great. I helped wipe glue off about 50 tiles ready for Dave to stick up.

Our anniversary is tomorrow, 15 years since our first date! I went out on a bit of a quest to buy Dave a pressie, I was thinking of getting him a picture but while I was having a look around a gallery Pear kicked me so hard he took my breath away and I had to grab a pole nearby - much to the shock of the guy who was showing me around, he thought I was going into labour! I made a quick exit stage left and got Dave some sweet treats instead.

Saturday 21st June

We celebrated our 15 year anniversary with an exchange of cards when we woke up. Dave also gave me some beautiful pink peonies that he knows I love so much and remind me of my wedding bouquet - so romantic and thoughtful of him. We did a bit more work on the tiling in the bathroom then escaped to Terre à Terre restaurant for a delicious lunch. I ate so much and yet still managed to squeeze in dessert. Pear was so good all day and didn't stick his 'tools' in me once - well at least not until we got home later.

Monday 23rd June

Busy day today, while Dave tiled I did the laundry and then wiped the grout off the wall he had finished. As per usual with all our experiences to date with tiling we had a wonky wall to contend with. Instead of a thin smear of adhesive Dave was getting through loads of the stuff. I was under strict instruction not to touch the tiles until they were totally dry as the adhesive was so thick they would just slide off.

I discovered a great company called 'Little Green Earthlets' and gave them a ring to discuss and order some washable nappies. I had done quite a bit of research online since visiting the Baby Expo and decided to go for the 'Mother-ease' ones in bamboo. With the help of a lovely lady on the phone Pear would hopefully have enough to take him right up to potty training. I came off the phone with my bank account severely dented but felt very pleased with myself.

In the afternoon we drove to 'Lili May' baby shop to pick up an Isofix for our car seat but they were out of stock so we ordered one instead - hopefully we would get it in time.

We did a big shop in Tesco, lots of healthy bits and pieces. We were so hungry by the time we got in so I rustled up a tasty stir-fry for dinner. We had been planning on getting an early night as Dave had an early start tomorrow. He was driving to Dover to sort out our property, as a tenant was moving in on Thursday and there were a few things that needed doing. I decided not to join him as I was finding car journeys really uncomfortable with my bump now.

Our early night didn't quite happen, and then Pear started kicking me loads. It felt as though he was on the diagonal again and sticking his arm or it could have been a leg out sideways. At one point I heard this odd and not particularly pleasant noise, a bit like when you crack your knuckles or back. Only it wasn't me that was cracking it was Pear!

Tuesday 24th June

Dave was up at 6 am while I got out of my nest at a far more civilised 10 am. I mooched about a bit then had a nice surprise when the doorbell went and Pears crib was delivered which was exciting.

I had lunch then went out for a wander and bumped into Cheryl so we had a quick drink and a chat. After I left Cheryl I went to Cath Kidston where I treated myself to a lovely white bag with colourful stars on it that I would call my 'birth bag' as opposed to a 'hospital bag' - where I was hoping I wouldn't have to go! I also got a gorgeous cowboy print change bag for Pear. It was lovely and had a matching change mat and bottle holder too. I went in Baby Gap and bought a pair of organic cotton, soft cream towelling trousers and a bodysuit. I think Pear knew I was buying things for him as he was so good all day - no 'tools' sticking in me or weird popping noises!

When I got home I mustered up some more energy to clean the windowsills in the bedroom which were filthy.

Tips and things to do

- Your baby is almost ready now and could drop into your birth canal at any time.

- Make sure you are eating healthily still and having around 2,400 calories a day - preferably from healthy sources and not entirely chocolate and cake!

- If you haven't done so already book your maternity leave.

- Practice any breathing techniques you have learnt in antenatal class.

- Learn how to swaddle your baby. We watched a great DVD called 'The Happiest Baby on the Block'. It showed in great detail how to swaddle a baby and it was amazing watching as previously screaming babies were instantly soothed by this. It made sense to us that after being in such a confined space that a baby would feel more secure tightly wrapped up. We were definitely going to try it out on Pear.

- Decide what type of nappies you plan to use. There are so many to choose from depending on what matters to you. I was determined to use washable nappies but was advised that it is best to use disposables for the first few days as the 'meconium' your baby will pass is like tar and not very easy to wash off your lovely new nappies. With the gift of hindsight I think I should have ordered less of the reusable nappies as although we used them for quite some time we did eventually succumb to disposables for convenience.

I finally pack a birth bag...

Wednesday 25th June

I had another great yoga class today and Pear even allowed me to get in most of the positions. After class I asked the other girls if they fancied meeting next week for a cup of tea and they all seemed up for it.

When I got home I found Dave snoozing on the sofa, exhausted from all the driving yesterday.

I spent the rest of the day doing housewifey things and in the evening caught up with my mum on the phone for a lovely chat.

Thursday 26th June

We had an appointment with the midwife first thing that went well; Pear was still in a good position despite my constant worry that he wasn't and he was also the right size...yippee!

It was such a beautiful day today so we decided to cut loose from the bathroom and spent some quality time together. It felt as though we hardly saw each other some days what with the never-ending D.I.Y. I knew it would be worth the hard graft to have the place up together before Pear arrived, but it was wonderful not to do any work and just hang out with each other.

Dave and I went to Mothercare to pick up some practical bits and pieces including a lovely blue and white polka dot change mat to put on the unit in the bathroom - once it was in! I also managed to find a lovely Elle Macpherson nursing bra that not only fitted nicely, was pink, lacy and reduced in price.

In the evening my stomach felt huge and went as hard as a bowling ball - I wondered if it was those 'Braxton Hicks' again. I thought they were practice contractions that I would feel, whereas I couldn't feel anything in particular, my stomach was just rock hard. I joked to Dave that I wasn't having a baby I was having a boulder instead!

To take my mind off the rock in my tummy I made a delicious gooseberry crumble and then Dave and I practiced our HypnoBirthing relaxation exercises for a couple of hours.

Friday 27th June

I didn't sleep too well last night as Pear was very active and my tummy felt so full and hard. Many of my pregnancy books said that the baby's movements got more restricted round now as the baby ran out of space but Pear was still managing to karate kick, dance and move furniture around!

I relaxed in the morning while Dave carried on with the tiles. I went for a little walk even though it was raining a bit and popped into Mothercare again. I bought Pear a lovely soft towel to wrap him in - I was getting so excited to meet him now.

I also got a couple of ceramic oil burners in a pound shop I was really pleased with. I was planning on getting some Frankincense and Lemongrass essential oils to burn while I was in labour. Every time we went to our HypnoBirthing class Karen was burning them, I loved the smell plus it would hopefully remind me of our classes and help me to relax.

In the evening I got a list of items that were suggested for your hospital/birth bag. I assembled lots of things on the bed and then packed them all in my new birth bag. Much as I was hoping to have Pear at home I realised it was sensible to have all these useful things in one place as I didn't want to be having to ask Dave to hunt around for them at the crucial moment. I felt a combination of excitement and satisfaction sorting it all out - I especially enjoyed folding up the little white bodysuits and imagining Pear wearing them sometime soon.

My list of things for my birth bag:

- *Birth plan/preferences*
- *Hypno notes (laminated so they don't get wet by the pool) & picture of the optimal position for birth*
- *Large brown towel*
- *Dressing gown*
- *Pyjamas and a nightie*
- *Slippers & socks*
- *Birth ball*
- *5 pairs of big knickers & sanitary towels*
- *Nursing bra and breast pads*
- *Toiletries in separate bag - toothbrush/paste, soap, moisturiser, make-up remover, eye cream, lip balm, face cloth, Arnica cream.*

- *Spare set of loose comfy clothes & extra t-shirt for Dave*
- *Water and snacks*
- *Oil burner & oils*
- *iPod - fully charged*
- *Phone with everyone's numbers in it & charger*
- *Camera*
- *CD of our favourite music and also classical harp music*
- *Pillows*
- *Massage oil*
- *Homeopathic birth kit*
- *Water spray and little battery operated fan*
- *Change for the car park and car seat (in case we had to go to hospital)*

For Pear I packed his change bag with the following:

- *2-3 white sleep suits and vests*
- *5-6 nappies real and eco-disposables*
- *Cotton wool*
- *Blanket*
- *Hat & cardigan*
- *Socks/booties*
- *Muslin squares*
- *Brown towel*

Saturday 28th June

I woke up with a bit of a sore throat today. While Dave started on the final wall in the bathroom I grouted all the tiles he had done so far. It was quite funny trying to manoeuvre myself into the corners while standing in the bath with my big bump.

It was a baking hot day and it felt doubly so sweltering away in the bathroom together. I made a salad for lunch and we escaped from the bathroom to eat it sat outside.

After lunch I went to 'JoJo Maman Bébé' where I bought another really comfy nursing bra which was a relief with my history of nightmare bra hunts.

Sunday 29th June

My throat was still sore so I decided to take it easy today and didn't get up to much. Dave was still at the tiling; I wondered if we would ever live somewhere that required just a couple of rows of tiles instead of the floor-to-ceiling epic we had going on. I ended up doing more grouting as all the tiles I did yesterday had dried with lots of air bubbles. After lunch I went through the cloth nappies we had bought and washed them all, as apparently that would make them more absorbent.

Monday 30th June

I felt so sorry for myself today as my throat was still sore plus my right kidney was really aching especially when I coughed.

We drove to the tip, again! Then the supermarket and M&S food hall where we bought some posh biscuits for any visitors we might have when Pear arrived.

After a healthy salad for lunch Dave returned to the bathroom for yet more tiling - we had got through so much adhesive it was unbelievable. I took it easy, read a book and had an early night. My throat was so sore I couldn't do my usual singing to Pear in the bath. It took ages to get off to sleep as I had such a horrible burning sensation in my throat.

Tuesday 1st July

I didn't feel as bad today as my throat was less sore but my kidney was still aching which wasn't good. Dave and I went out to do a few errands and we got a gorgeous grobag for Pear to sleep in from Cath Kidston with a cowboy print on, the same as his change bag. I bought a couple of great breastfeeding tops in 'JoJo Maman Bébé' - they were cap sleeved with a crossover style that was very flattering.

We had salad for lunch - I was quite pleased with how healthy I had managed to be as I thought I would be craving all manner of strange things. I did succumb to treating us to a homemade vegan cheesecake that was totally scrummy. After dinner I got second wind and did some laundry and washed the kitchen floor that was a bit sticky from my cooking. I found it hard to get to sleep - no heartburn but my tummy just felt so full it was difficult to get in a comfy position. I started each day off OK but by the evening my ribs and internal organs all seemed to be in different locations to usual making breathing tricky.

Tips and things to do

- Your baby practices breathing movements this week and will turn towards a bright light.

- Once your baby drops into the birth canal you should find eating and breathing easier. If your baby hasn't dropped yet - Pear hadn't at this point - try to eat your main meal at lunchtime and snack between then and your evening meal, which is probably best being smaller to help with the lack of space you have between your ribs and bump.

- If your baby does drop you may find it more difficult to walk, or waddle as I was at this time!

- Pamper yourself - watch a film, get your nails done, go out for a meal with your partner or a friend - spend time doing whatever you enjoy most.

- Have fun with a bit of retail therapy buying some essentials for your baby. I have listed some of my favourite retailers at the end of this book.

WEEK 38

Perineal massage!

Wednesday 2nd July

I did my yoga class and afterwards Cheryl, me and another girl from class called Sara went for tea and cake together. We had a great chat and I was so happy to be making new friends. Fortunately I felt so much better today, so I could resume singing to Pear in the bath and talking to Dave which I had missed. My intercostals on the right were still painful from coughing and blowing my nose so much.

I had been reading in my HypnoBirthing book and online about the importance of having a perineal massage. According to my book it was good to do it every night between now and the birth. I bought some sweet almond oil and asked Dave to do it for me and that was when it all went a bit wrong. Now whoever decided to call it a perineal massage - which implies something pleasant and relaxing when actually it was more of a perineum stretch - was obviously having a bit of a joke! After dimming the lights in the bedroom, burning my new essential oils and playing some lovely relaxing harp music I had bought recently the moment was ruined when Dave announced he couldn't find my perineum.

I ended up getting a bit tearful as I felt like I had failed at a really important piece of homework. Plus it was a bit of a worry that if Dave couldn't find it how on earth was Pear going to get out!

It took ages to get off to sleep as my back was still hurting and I just couldn't find a comfortable position.

Thursday 3rd July

We had a lovely day today; went to see the midwife who was a different one to usual, but very nice. She booked us in for a homebirth which was so exciting and also told us Pear was in the perfect position...hooray! My blood pressure was a bit higher than usual but I thought that was because I was bubbling with excitement and she didn't seem concerned about it.

We spent the afternoon doing some shopping; we bought a couple of white cotton sheets for Pear's crib, another grobag that was a lightweight summer one from 'JoJo Maman Bébé' with a duck egg blue background and big white stars on it - very cute. We also got Pear his first toy - a wonderfully soft, blue elephant that had a very relaxing jangle/chime to it when you shook it. BHS was having a sale and we also bought a couple of luxurious dark brown towels - a bath sheet size one for me and a hand towel to wrap little Pear in when he was born. I felt very clever and practical buying brown as any stains should a) not really show and b) wash out easily.

Friday 4th July

I woke up today with such a runny nose still and the muscles around my back sore from yet another night of coughing. I didn't feel ill but was finding it a bit difficult breathing as I was so congested.

The boiler had been playing up so we got our trusty plumber, Paul, to come and take a look. Shortly after he left I could smell gas which must have been bad if I could smell it with my blocked nose. Paul came back and made sure everything was safe. We could do with a new boiler as this one was antiquated but the timing wasn't great. Paul fixed our old one as best he could so we would just have to keep our fingers crossed it didn't break down. It wouldn't be great having a homebirth with no hot water and I didn't think I could last without my nightly soak in the bath.

Again my tummy was solid as a rock in the evening.

Saturday 5th July

It was another lovely sunny day today. Dave was still tiling but hopefully on the home straight. I made pizza for lunch and some flapjacks I had a fancy for. I just couldn't wait for the bathroom to be done so we could put all our toiletries in our new units and finally pack all the tools away. Everywhere was so dusty and needed a good clean but it was impossible to start while Dave was still creating more mess. I hoped all the D.I.Y. got completed and that Dave and I could spend some quality time together before Pear joined us. I shocked myself when I measured my stomach and it was a whopping 40 inches!

Sunday 6th July

I didn't sleep particularly well last night as my bump was so big now it was putting pressure on my ribs causing them to ache. We got up at 10 am and Dave hit the bathroom again. I was hoping he would get onto putting the sink in today but Wimbledon was on TV and he spent 5 hours watching that instead, bless him. I really hoped Pear would hang in there until Dave finished, but saying that I didn't want to go too overdue! I was so tired I took a bit of a nap but for some strange reason I kept startling myself awake again. In the end I got up and joined Dave watching TV. I tried my best to get him enthused about putting some of his tool collection away but the tennis came back on so I gave up in the end. It was so frustrating as in the past I would've just got on with things myself, but the pile of tools in the hallway were just too awkward and heavy and I didn't want to do my back in. Instead I caught up with some paperwork and later my groin started aching on the right side.

Monday 7th July

We went through what was becoming a bit of a ritual for us of filling the car with rubbish for the tip. It took so long so we had lunch and went to the tip via the parking permit office. I didn't enjoy the car ride one bit as my tummy felt so slopped about and every bump seemed to set Pear wiggling around. The good news was that we had finally got to the top of the list for a parking permit. Despite wanting to have a homebirth I felt relieved to know that at least now the car would be in the same street as where we lived and not some 20 minute walk away. By the time we got to the tip it was shut so we left everything in the car overnight and hoped it wasn't too stinky in the morning.

Tips and things to do

- Your baby's first bowel movement known as 'meconium' is gathering in his or her intestine.

- As it gets more difficult to find a comfy position to sleep in at night try to take some naps during the day when you're not feeling as full.

- Massaging your perineum (the area between you vagina and rectum) is supposed to help prevent tearing during birth. I can't say it was the most pleasant thing to do but as with many things the more practice the better. Just take it gently and maybe ask your partner to do it for you while you practice your relaxation and breathing exercises.

- If you are planning on having your baby at home it's a good idea to collect up all your old towels and bed linen to use. Where we had been decorating for so long we had a massive assortment of old sheets and duvets we used as dust sheets that came in handy. The brown towels I purchased were particularly good as they felt luxurious but my choice of colour meant I didn't need to worry about spoiling them.

Birth pool in a box...

Wednesday 9th July

It was yucky weather today and I nearly didn't go to
yoga. In the end I decided to haul myself out in the
drizzle and was so glad I did as the class was lovely.
Afterwards I invited Cheryl back to ours for tea and
toast which was nice. I didn't venture out again for the
rest of the day as it was too wet, instead I hit the phone
sorting a few things out. I had been toying for ages with
the possibility of hiring a birth pool and decided to ring
our local active birth centre to find out some more info.
The lady I spoke to was surprised I had left it so late
and said she had already hired all her available pools
out...darn! I went back online and came across a site
called 'The Good Birth Company' that specialised in
birth pools. I read up on one of their products called
'Birth Pool in a Box' and for a reasonable price you got
your own birth pool with a liner and pump. I went ahead
and placed an order, asking for an extra liner so we could
inflate the pool before the birth and have a little practice.
Dave and I spent ages with the tape measure working
out where would be best to put it in our tiny living room.
I was a bit worried that with the weight of me and the

water that I might well go through the ceiling but Dave assured me that if we put it near to the wall the load should be spread over the most stable part of the building...fingers crossed!

I also telephoned the lovely doula, Samsara we met at the Baby Expo and she was still available. We arranged for her to come over tomorrow to meet us properly at home and if it all went well we would go ahead and book her.

I was a bit worried about Pear in the evening as he didn't move around much when I was singing to him in the bath - maybe he was sleeping, he was probably getting quite bored by my repertoire of songs by now.

Thursday 10th July

Pear made up for his lack of movement Wednesday evening by wiggling around all night long; at least I knew he was OK.

I went to the hairdressers today - my hair looked much better, but I was there ages and ended up so hot and flustered. I got to a point when I just wanted to go home and didn't even care if the hairdresser hadn't dried my hair.

By the time I got in I was so tired and hungry. After a bite to eat I felt much better and the rest of the evening was great. Samsara came over and we got along so well with her. She was such a fountain of information and although we didn't have any spare cash available I knew having her with us at Pear's birth would make me feel so much more confident, so we went for it and booked her.

Friday 11th July

My lovely friend Amanda came to visit us today. It was a nice sunny day and we had lunch together in Infinity

Cafe and a good old chin-wag. She left to catch her train home at 3.30 pm and I went to our estate agents to get a solicitor pack and pay a deposit for the upcoming auction of our freehold, which still landed the same day as my due date.

Dave and I went to pick up some drawers and bedside cupboards that we ordered some time ago. We were disappointed upon opening the packaging to discover that they were quite badly damaged and not even what we had ordered. We had been so excited about the prospect of finally having proper storage in our bedroom that Dave had already taken the old shelves down in readiness so we were now in even more of a muddle than before.

Dave finished putting the bathroom sink in at 1.30 am and I stayed up to put away our toiletries which was very exciting.

Saturday 12th July

I slept so much better last night - usually I went to bed, woke up at 1.30 am hungry and got up to eat a yoghurt or two, then woke again at 3 am, 5 am and 7 am mostly to sleepwalk to the loo. Last night I did go to bed late but slept till 4 am and only woke up again at 7 am so that was a major improvement. Although I figured all this night waking was good practice for when Pear was born.

Dave and I walked up the high street to buy blinds for the living room windows - a must as we planned on giving birth there and I didn't want to shock the neighbours!

Sunday 13th July

Dave and I went to Sainsbury's; well Dave drove the car and I walked and met him there as I just couldn't cope with all the bumps and bends in the road. After lunch Dave spent the rest of the day cleaning grout off all the tiles I'd done. It took him ages and I did get a bit stressed out about it as I didn't think I had done that bad a job, but saying that it looked great when he'd finished. I made us a lovely roast dinner while Dave sealed the bath in.

Monday 14th July

The post arrived this morning and Dave said that all the neighbours would now know what we were up to as my birth pool arrived in a big parcel with 'Birth Pool in a Box' in huge writing on every side, how funny!

We thought we would have a go at blowing up the pool until we realised I had forgotten to order a hosepipe or connectors, doh! So Dave went to Screwfix to see if he could get some there. He returned with a huge roll of garden hosepipe at a bargain price.

The evening ended in tears when Dave started to build our new crib and we found that the company had sent us the wrong one. It was all just too much for me and I cried into some tissue, if Pear arrived early not only didn't we have a crib for him, we couldn't even put him in a drawer as a temporary measure as we didn't have them either!

Tuesday 15th July

After all the drama of the wrong drawers and crib Dave was my hero and spent today sorting it all out. He came home triumphant with the right drawers this time and he had even managed to get the baby shop to loan us a Moses basket and sheets as a back-up in case the new crib didn't arrive before Pear did - what a star!

The stand for the Moses basket was a nightmare to assemble, it took Dave an hour and he was usually brilliant at reading dodgy instructions. I lined the drawers with some wallpaper we had left over and put Dave's clothes in them.

In the evening Samsara came over again to chat about our birth plan and generally get to know us. We gave her copies of our birth preferences and the terminology that HypnoBirthing uses for her to become familiar with. She was lovely with a calm, confident and very caring disposition. Both Dave and I got a really good vibe from her, she was able to answer so many questions we had and also gave us lots of good tips and bits of advice. I knew in my heart that she was the perfect person for us to have with us, on what would be the most amazing day of our lives.

Tips and things to do

- Most of the lanugo that was covering your baby has gone by now and his or her lungs are maturing.

- The average baby weighs just over 7 pounds at this point.

- You may feel clumsy as your baby settles into your pelvis.

- Take it easy this week; spend some quality time with your partner.

- It is a good idea to assemble any furniture, crib, birth pool etc. to check you have all the pieces. We wished we had unpacked the box containing our crib sooner, as it did cause an unnecessary bit of stress we could have done without!

- Practice putting the car seat in. You don't want to be fiddling around with a new born for the lack of a bit of practice beforehand.

- Get a last trip in to the hairdresser's for a while. I was glad I did as I feel so much better with a freshly highlighted head of hair. It was a long time once Pear was born before I went again.

We test drive the pool...

Wednesday 16th July

I had such a good sleep last night - only woke at 3.30 am and 5 am and didn't even get out of bed the second time.

Yoga today was with a different teacher, which was a bit disappointing as I had bought some gorgeous sunflowers for Dom as a thank you just in case I didn't make next week, as it was my due date.

It was the wedding anniversary of our Brighton blessing so we celebrated with a lovely meal at Food for Friends. Afterwards we went to Mothercare where I bought a couple more pairs of leggings as mine had gone a bit strange in the wash and were ridiculously short in the leg.

The highlight of the day was when we test drove our birth pool, it was amazing. Dave did something clever with the hosepipe so that the water came out lovely and hot straight into the pool, and as it cooled he just added more. We both hopped in - I hadn't felt so light in ages and it was great being able to submerge my entire body, as in the bath my boobs were always above water. We stayed in the pool for ages, Dave got me a wine glass of water - well, I could always pretend, and we watched Neighbours and Home and Away, how decadent!

To empty the pool out Dave used the rest of the hosepipe and had it running from the pool, down the stairs, over the bathroom door and down the loo - my hubby is nothing if not inventive! It was so good; I wished we'd bought it weeks ago as I would have made so much use of it. We had got another liner for the birth but until then this one was fine to keep in the pool, so I would be in it every night until Pear arrived.

Thursday 17th July

My friend Richard rang and we had such a good catch up and a giggle, he promised to visit soon. By the time I got off the phone I realised it was nearly time for my appointment with the midwife so I power-waddled up there with Dave. It went really well, she listened to Pears heartbeat and checked he was still in a good position, which he was. She also checked my blood pressure and said it was lower than the last appointment which was a relief.

The rest of the day was spent tiding up - at last everything was coming together and I felt so happy and contented.

Friday 18th July

Poor Dave did his back in - he was trying to put tarpaulin under the pool and twisted it while moving a large pot plant. I came upstairs to find him lying on the floor on top of metres of blue tarpaulin! I felt terrible he had hurt himself; hopefully it would ease of soon.

In the afternoon Cheryl came by to see us, I showed her our wedding pictures and birth pool - she had ordered the same one as well, although her flat was huge so she would have lots more space.

In the evening Dave and I relaxed in the pool which was great for my bump and his back. As I looked across the room I noticed that the wallpaper was starting to peel off where it had got so steamy…whoops!

Saturday 19th July

Dave was up first and made me a delicious smoothie, recently I'd a craving for cherries so we had been blending frozen cherries, soya milk and banana, delicious! Dave was treating me so well and was being amazing especially as I knew his back was still playing him up - I am so lucky to have him as my hubby.

I listened to my HypnoBirthing affirmations - I had been very good listening to them every morning and the 'Rainbow Relaxation' every night, so I really hoped they would help.

We went up the high street to buy a little plastic step or stool as I was positively dangerous getting in and out the pool - the wall of which was higher than my inner leg which made manoeuvring really difficult. I usually ended up getting stuck with Dave either pushing or pulling me depending on whether I was on my way in or way out.

Sunday 20th July

Dave was a man on a mission today, while Pear and I lazed in the bath (naughty but nice!) Dave did the tip, the supermarket and put the last of our pictures up - it was finishing touches like that that make the flat feel really homely and ours.

We went to The Pavilion gardens for a walk/waddle - there were lots of babies with their mums and dads enjoying the day and we got so excited thinking that we would be a family soon. We couldn't wait to take Pear out with us, introduce him to the world as well as all the things we wanted to do with him.

I cooked a tasty veggie roast in the evening but ate a bit too much. Dave read a lovely balloon relaxation and deepening exercise from our HypnoBirthing book to me while I relaxed, like a beached whale. I found it hard to breath I was just so full of baby.

Monday 21st July
I did my usual 1 am, 3 am, 5 am and 7 am awakenings - I was going to be glad when Pear was born and my bladder could have a bit more space again.

It was a beautiful day today; Paul returned to replace a part on our boiler, unfortunately rather like when you tinker with an old car it had a bit of a knock on effect and now we could only get hot water when the safety valve was off.

Dave and I made the most of the sun and the fact that everything was pretty much finished in the flat to take a relaxing walk to the beach.

Tuesday 22nd July
We were up early today as Paul came by to check the boiler again. He had been planning on washing it through with acid or something that sounded a bit harsh. He said he had been lying in bed worrying about our situation and thought it was best not to do anything else just in case it made matters worse, as at the moment it seemed to be working OK.

I had booked us a refresher session with Karen just to give us a little boost before the big day, which was supposedly tomorrow - although Karen said it was not so much a 'due date' but more of a 'guess date' and that most babies came later. Our session was brilliant, we were there for about 3 hours going over the relaxation exercises and asking her questions. She also lent us a couple of DVDs to watch.

Afterwards we were famished so we popped into M&S for some food. They had a cafe but as there were no vegan options we picked up some salad, crisps and water from their store. I was hungry and exhausted but there was nowhere to sit down so Dave suggested we sat in the cafe - after all we had purchased the food from the same place he reasoned. Now I had a bit of a bad feeling about it but let him take charge and the next minute this horrible 'jobs worth' of a woman came over and gave us a right telling off. I felt my cheeks redden and eyes fill with tears as she talked to us as though we were 5 years old. Worse still were the sympathetic looks other customers were giving us and doubtless thinking, 'What a mean old cow can't she see that woman is about to give birth, give her a break!'

We went to the baby shop to pick up the replacement crib but it was still missing some important parts to attach the wheels. In the end Dave assembled it without them and I put the sheets on - so we were all ready.

It seemed strange lying in bed later looking across at the gorgeous crib and thinking that someday soon a little person would be in it.

Tips and things to do

- This may be your last week of your pregnancy - or not. It is such an exciting time but you may also be feeling a bit impatient and ready to meet your baby.

Enjoy these last few days as a couple by doing things together.

- By this week the average baby is about 20 inches long and 7 $\frac{1}{2}$ pounds. I entertained myself for ages with a tape measure trying to imagine how on earth a 20 inch baby was in my tummy and more so how he was going to get out!

- Get your baby's crib ready and wash bed linen in a non-biological soap.

- Stock up on food. If you are planning on having a homebirth make sure you have lots of bread in the freezer, tea, coffee and biscuits on hand to keep your midwives, doula and husband going - oh yes and you of course!

Cole Jayden - aka
Pear makes his entrance...

Wednesday 23rd July

It was my due/guess date today and also the day of the auction of our freehold. I went to yoga - it was the last session before the summer break and would definitely be my last class. I managed not to give birth during it and had a great time. The sunflowers I had bought Dom were still looking good so I gave them to her at the end of the lesson. It was strange to say goodbye to the other girls in the class knowing that the next time we saw each other we would all be mummies.

When I got home Nick was with Dave as we had enlisted his help with the auction. He had very kindly offered to go on our behalf, as it didn't seem a great idea me being there. I get quite excited at auctions at the best of times and would most likely go into labour and miss our lot! As it looked as though Pear wouldn't be joining us Dave went to the auction with Nick. They returned a few hours later with the news that we had lost out to a millionaire who collected freeholds. He paid far more than our limit so there wasn't much the boys could do short of holding the guy's arm down.

It was all such an anti-climax we just hoped he was a nice freeholder who wouldn't try to make money out of us as we didn't have any!

We went to the beach, Dave and Nick went in the sea while I sat in the sun until I got too hot.

Later I told dad all about the auction, he couldn't believe it - well it was another thing to put in the ****it bucket!

Thursday 24th July

It was the hottest day of the year so far and so we just relaxed until 3 pm when I had an appointment with my midwife.

The rest of the day was terrible. Instead of my usual lovely, chilled-out midwife Ruth, I had a different lady. The appointment started OK with her telling us Pear was 1/5th engaged which was good. She then took my blood pressure and told me it was too high at 140/90 and that as it was my 3rd high-ish reading she wouldn't be doing her job properly if she ignored it. I tried saying to her that strictly speaking it was actually only the 2nd high result as I'd had an extra unofficial appointment just to check Pear's position. She wasn't having any of that and started scaremongering me about the chances of me getting pre-eclampsia. While I was in the toilet peeing on a stick Dave explained to her that we were planning a Hypno Birth and could she refrain from any negative stories. That was like waving a red rag to a bull; as when I returned she started telling me birth stories that frankly were quite upsetting. She made it clear, in no uncertain terms that if I didn't get checked out at the hospital I was being reckless with both mine and Pear's health. I asked her to take my blood pressure again, thinking that as we'd been rushing to get to the appointment and as it was such a hot day that maybe that could have had an effect too. It was a fraction higher than the previous reading - most likely because by now I was feeling quite upset and stressed out. I told her about my relaxation CD and she said that it wasn't possible to lower your own blood pressure (something I was sure wasn't true).

Dave and I were desperate to get out of the place and sat on the wall outside, me almost crying and Dave feeling annoyed at how brusque she had been with us. I made a couple of phone calls to Karen and Samsara to ask them what they thought we should do. Just speaking to them I felt a lot calmer and they both were of the opinion that I should get checked out, but to stay firm on the fact that we were having a homebirth and didn't want any medical intervention at this stage to bring on labour.

At the hospital we were taken to a room with the most amazing view of the pier and the sun shimmering on the sea. I zoned out listening to my 'Rainbow Relaxation' on my iPod and by the time the nurse came to take my blood pressure it had gone down to something over 63! So my CD did work. I got all stressed out again when the nurse said she would be back in half an hour and if it stayed the same I could go home - no pressure there then! When she returned I had a severe case of performance anxiety and it rose to 146/92! I realised that if I wanted to go home that I had to calm myself down so I just closed my eyes and kept listening to my HypnoBirthing relaxation and breathed deeply. The next time she took my blood pressure I'd got it down to 140/86 and the nurse said we could go home but to return on Monday.

I was so glad to get out of the hospital; by now it was gone 6 pm and we had left home at 2.40 pm so we were starving, hot and tired. Once we had eaten I went through my pregnancy bible to read up on blood pressure and pre-eclampsia. It said that during pregnancy readings up to 140/90 were fairly common so I felt a bit better.

Friday 25th July

We relaxed in the morning recovering from the stressy day we had yesterday.

After lunch I went to Neal's Yard and bought a Homeopathic Birth Kit, an empty bottle with a spray so I could mix some oils to use at Pear's birth and some Emergency Essence (a Bush Flower Rescue Remedy). I could have done with some of it at the hospital yesterday.

We got yet more food at Sainsbury's - just what Dave could carry. Every shop we did we thought would be the last before Pear's birthday and then we ended up eating it all and needing to buy more.

I found it tricky getting in a comfy position to sleep, in the end I lay on top of the duvet with a sheet over me, propped up with lots of pillows.

Saturday 26th July

In the morning we had a bit of a smooch session in the hopes of encouraging Pear to make his entrance - we really couldn't wait to meet him now.

We went to 'JoJo Maman Bébé' and got a great sling that Samsara had recommended to us. It was basically a long piece of fabric with instructions to make several different styles of 'wearing' your baby that were suitable from birth to 2 years. The lady in the shop gave us a demo with a doll and made it look easy, so hopefully we would get along with it.

I got ingredients to make a curry - yet another tip from our HypnoBirthing class that was supposed to help encourage labour to start.

Sunday 27th July

I woke with a sinking feeling in my tummy worrying about going back to hospital tomorrow to be monitored. I was sure stressing about it was making my blood pressure even higher.

I busied myself with little jobs all day in an attempt to take my mind off it and did lots of relaxation exercises before bed.

Monday 28th July

I was so nervous about going into hospital today; I could feel our dream of having a homebirth slipping away.

Dave and I went to a different level at the hospital from last time, which was more like a doctor's waiting room. We saw this lovely man - who I thought was head of the midwifery department. As I recounted how we had been treated by the midwife at my last appointment he was quite shocked and said he would definitely be following it up. I found myself getting tearful as I relived the horrible time we had on Thursday. I am sensitive at the best of times but whenever I get sympathy I now find it impossible not to cry. A nurse came to take my blood pressure and as expected it was really high. They put Pear on a monitor for half an hour and thankfully he was fine; it was just me that needed sorting out. I kept listening to my HypnoBirthing 'Rainbow Relaxation' again and again - trying to zone out of the nightmare.

They took my blood to test and checked my urine for protein which was given the all clear so that was good. We stayed in the hospital for a lengthy 5 hours in total. I managed to get my blood pressure down...Yay! And then my blood test came back showing no markers for pre-eclampsia... double Yay! I felt so relieved and started to think that things were looking up until another doctor came to see me and started counting how many days I was past my 'due/guess date'. She told me I needed to have my baby by the 3rd of August - no pressure there then! She was also keen to give me a membrane sweep which we politely but firmly declined, we still wanted to do things naturally and our own way. I was so thankful for all the things Karen taught us, I felt pretty certain that if we hadn't done the course we would have been talked out of a homebirth and into a membrane sweep by now.

We finally got home, hungry, hot and flustered but glad to be out of the hospital. Dave bought some fresh pineapple - another thing that was supposed to help with encouraging labour to start and we had the most amazing sex ever...

Tuesday 29th July

I woke up at 1 am feeling that something may be happening baby-wise! Hard to explain but every 15-20 minutes I had a sensation not unlike before my period usually starts. I was so excited I wanted to wake Dave up but he was sleeping soundly and looked very cosy so I resisted the temptation. Instead I wandered around the flat eating yoghurts until 4 am when I couldn't contain my excitement anymore and woke him up. We both had a moment of, 'Yippee it's really happening!' Dave started to time my surges and they seemed to be quite regular and gradually got closer. At 6.30 am Dave rang Samsara while I had a bath. She arrived at 8 am by which time I was in the bedroom relaxing listening to my Hypno CD and burning my frankincense and lemongrass oils. I found that one minute I would be chatting away to her and Dave then a surge would come along - I now really understood why they were referred to as surges and not contractions. To me a contraction implied almost a sensation of doing a sit-up or of the muscles tensing whereas what I was experiencing was more like a surge. Not painful but very powerful, almost like a surge of electricity or power running through my body that I had no control over. I found I just had to focus totally on it and once it had past I was chatting again, eating travel sweets and more yoghurt! Some of the surges were strong and I found myself grabbing hold of Pear's crib, which without its wheels was very sturdy. Sometimes I knelt or squatted on the floor on a little nest of cushions Samsara had made for me. I also found great relief when she held a hot water bottle in the small of my back as I lay on my side on the bed. Every time a surge came along I did my breathing exercises, and when they passed I felt so relaxed and just kept thinking, 'That one is over, there won't be another the same'. At times I found myself sitting on the toilet with my hands in the pockets of my dressing gown hooked on the back of the door. When the surges were particularly strong it was really comforting to hang off it with my face buried in the lovely soft robe.

Things carried on like this for some time then we moved upstairs to get in our birth pool, which was wonderful. By 4 pm I was getting strong surges and was in my own little zone listening to my CD which I had been playing constantly - it must have been driving

Dave and Samsara crazy but I loved it. As time passed I thought it was odd that no midwife had turned up yet. I started to feel a bit concerned about it as by now I felt ready to give birth. At one point Samsara whispered in my ear, 'Try not to have him till the midwife gets here sweetheart.'

Thankfully a lovely midwife did arrive and was brilliantly 'hands off' just as we had requested. I had already decided I didn't want to be examined and told how many centimetres I was dilated. I figured that once the process had begun our baby and my body would do things in their own time and I couldn't see the point of being told measurements, it was just another thing to worry about and break my concentration from the job in hand! The midwife was so respectful of my wishes and just monitored Pear from time to time which was reassuring as she kept saying, 'Yes he's fine'. Dave was absolutely amazing - he was with me in the pool and supported me from behind. As the surges intensified I found myself pushing down hard on him and after-wards apologizing profusely for hurting his back. It was such a loving, relaxing environment - sometimes I held Samsara's hand, sometimes the midwife's and I didn't think I had ever felt so serene and looked after.

As the time passed and the surges grew closer and stronger my overwhelming feeling physically was one of wanting to do a poo - which was totally not how I had expected it to feel! The midwife explained that this was because of the position Pear was in as he was pushing on my sphincter muscles as he made his way down - little rascal! The surges started to come in 4's and it took all my focus and strength to breath through them. At one point the midwife asked if I would like to touch Pear's head - it was amazing and a real boost that he would soon be with us. I had never truly appreciated before the sense of touch alone. His little head felt so soft and downy and later when I heard the midwife say, 'He's bald!' I knew without seeing him that she was wrong as I had felt his gorgeous hair.

The second midwife arrived and I made a visit to the toilet where my surges were so strong that I was literally hanging off my dressing gown I was quite surprised I didn't rip the pockets or the hooks off the back of the door! When the surge passed my arms felt so full of lactic acid, as if I had been lifting very heavy bags.

I got back in the pool and for a while the surges intensified and became closer. I could hear my voice but it didn't sound like me - I went from sounding a bit like an extra from an adult movie to making a more guttural noise as things got harder - so for any neighbours who hadn't seen our birth pool being delivered they must have known by now what we were up too!

At this point the midwives became like my very own cheerleading squad, urging me to keep going even after I had lost the desire to keep breathing down. Pear had got caught on my cervix which was causing a see-sawing effect I felt he had moved down to my first knuckle but I couldn't seem to get him any further. At this point I felt really tired so Samsara kept giving me travel sweets and water which helped with my energy levels. Everyone was so supportive especially my wonderful Dave.

I got out of the pool for a while and had some time on the sofa. I was examined, my blood pressure was taken and so was Pear's - we were both OK but I did start feeling that if I didn't make progress soon I may have to go to hospital - even though no-one actually said this to me. By now it was 6 pm; I was getting quite tired between surges and felt limp, as though I was on drugs although all I had running through my blood stream was travel sweets and vegan yoghurt. Amazingly for me, at no time did I feel scared or panicky; it must have been all those lovely endorphins and oxytocin coursing through my body.

Eventually one of the midwives suggested that I got out of the pool and that maybe walking up and down the stairs would help - was she kidding me? The last thing I felt like doing was walking up and down stairs! She then noticed that the temperature had dropped quite considerably in the pool - of all times the boiler chose to pack in now!

Once they had managed to get me out the pool I did find walking downstairs was great for gravity. When we got to the bedroom I had a bit of an eureka moment when I realised that I needed to make my 4 surges stretch to 7 or 8 if I was going to succeed in helping our baby to be born soon. By now I was calling to Pear how much I loved him and would he PLEASE come out! Just a minute before 7 pm Samsara grabbed a mirror from the wall in the hallway and with me squatting on our nest, Dave behind me and Samsara and the midwives in front, we all witnessed the miracle of Pear being born. It was AWESOME. I was so glad for Samsara's quick thinking as I was able to see Pear's head then body slip out like a dream. We had him straight on my tummy and he just looked right at me and we fell in love instantly. He was amazing, so alert and perfect. His colour came really quickly and we just cuddled him. The midwife asked me to push a little to get the placenta out - I had thought this part of the proceedings would be really difficult and horrible as I got queasy about most things - instead it was easy and fascinating at the same time seeing just how large it was. The midwife checked it was all complete, which it was and we waited until Pear's umbilical cord stopped pulsing before it was cut. Once again we surprised ourselves when Dave was asked if he would like to do the honours and he said yes...perfect. Pear tried to do the breast crawl and made it to my boob but didn't latch on; he was too busy looking around. One of the midwives remarked how alert he was - this was a trait Karen was always saying HypnoBirthing babies had.

Dave, Pear and I moved to the bed and I was checked down below. The midwife said I had torn a muscle or something inside - most probably when they had tried to help stretch me towards the end. I was given the choice of having stitches or letting it heal naturally which would take slightly longer. As I had got this far naturally I decided to opt out of having stitches as I just wanted to be with my baby and Dave. It was quite funny as one of the midwives asked me, 'How heavy do you think your baby is?' What did she think I was a human scale? I just guessed 7lbs 7oz as that was how much I weighed when I was born. Surprisingly he weighed a whopping 9lbs 5oz - no wonder he was playing see-saw for so long.

Dave and I were over the moon, we found we couldn't stop looking at our gorgeous baby - Cole Jayden.

The midwives left, Samsara stayed - she tidied everything, did our washing-up and put some laundry on, earning herself forever with us the title 'Angel Samsara'. I took a lovely bath with Cole; he lay on my tummy and appeared to enjoy the experience.

After the bath Samsara dressed Cole for us in a lovely white vest bodysuit and swaddled him in a blue cellular blanket. It was wonderful to have her expert advice on hand as Dave and I hadn't looked beyond the birth so we didn't have a clue how to dress or wrap a baby! She finally left us in bed with tea, toast and marmalade - never had tea and toast tasted as good.

After Samsara had gone we settled in for the night - Cole looked like a little angel in his swaddling and had the most amazing eyes. We laid him in his crib right next to us and he kept looking at us all night long and us at him. He seemed pretty content to be in our world and we felt so blessed to have experienced what we had today and to be a family at last.

Tips and things to do

- You may be feeling a bit anxious that your baby still hasn't made their entrance yet but try to relax and not worry - I know it's easier said than done!

- Busy yourself with any little jobs, such as preparing your baby's crib and sorting out their clothes. I got so excited folding all the tiny little outfits and wondering when my little fella would arrive to wear them.

- There are lots of natural things you can do to help promote labour and I think we tried all of them. Fresh pineapple, curry, a long walk and my favourite - some sex - certainly worked for us!

- Until your baby arrives take time to relax each day, if you have a birth pool or bath they are both nice ways to take the weight off your body.

- If you have the opportunity to practice dressing or changing a nappy on any of your friend's babies then do. Both Dave and I were incredibly cautious about putting anything over Cole's head and don't even get me started on the nappy changing - 'totally clueless' are the words that spring to mind!

- Make sure you have some bottled water and energy giving snacks that you can nibble on during labour. I had bought some delicious flapjacks but found that during my surges I just couldn't concentrate on breathing and chewing at the same time and ended up spitting it out...nice! I found travel sweets and yoghurt the easiest things to eat washed down with lots of water. Ask your partner or birth companion beforehand to remind you to drink water frequently to stay hydrated, as in all the excitement it is easy to forget to eat and drink.

- Whether you are planning a hospital, birthing unit or homebirth, have any home comforts to hand for the big day. Items such as an iPod with your favourite music or relaxation exercises on. If you like essential oils make sure you have packed the burner, oils and matches. Also if you are giving birth during the summer you may want to have a small fan or water spritzer as well.

- If you remember, ask a friend or your partner to buy a newspaper from the day of your baby's birth to keep for him or her in your keepsake box.

- Have your camera at the ready to give to the midwife or your doula for that all important picture of the three of you together as a family at last!

The first few days
as a new family...

After a bit of sleep Dave and I started texting and telephoning family and friends with our fantastic news. The next few days were a blur of family coming to see Cole interspersed with frequent visits from the midwives or health visitor. We had planned on having a 'baby moon' but it was hard to stick to as our family were understandably so excited to meet Cole straight away and we were equally keen to show him off to all the special people in our lives.

When we were talking about everything we had experienced Dave made a confession to me - the reason that the midwives had arrived quite late in the proceedings was that he had actually turned the first midwife away! To explain, at around 9 am the door bell had rung and when Dave went to answer it he instantly recognised the midwife who had upset us during my last appointment. He then made the brave and right decision for us to turn her away. He later said that he knew if he had let her in she would have been the wrong person to have at our baby's birth and things could have turned out so differently for us. I was so grateful to Dave for being protective of us; he truly demonstrated what we had learned in our HypnoBirthing classes that the husband could be a silverback gorilla. When Karen found out she was most impressed that Dave had taken so much of what she'd said on-board and he is now her star pupil!

I did experience difficulties breastfeeding which surprised me as I had a pre-conceived idea of it being easy and something that would come naturally to me. So much emphasis was placed on the birth itself and I didn't recall anyone mentioning that breastfeeding could be painful or the joys of the dreaded mastitis!

Cole was totally mesmerising and as every day passed we found that we were learning so much about him and more importantly he was teaching us how to be parents. Dave and I were a strong team taking it in turns to change nappies, comfort, cuddle and adore this wonderful little person who had blessed our lives so completely.

For weeks we remained in our own little bubble, floating around in a semi-sleep deprived state of total bliss. We were so happy if a little overwhelmed to have finally made it to the amazing place Samsara introduced us to and always spoke so fondly of - 'Baby Land' - and we were ready to embrace everything that comes with being parents and a family at last.

Tips and things to do

- Huge congratulations to you and welcome to the best club in the world 'Motherhood' that exists in that magical place I like to call 'Baby Land'.

- You are probably feeling so many emotions at this time ranging from elation at finally meeting your gorgeous baby, to confusion as to what to do next! Don't worry you are not alone there. Dave and I had not wanted to tempt fate by reading too much about impending parenthood and did feel quite ill-equipped as to how best to look after our new baby. From how many layers to place on him in his crib, to how best to position him for feeding. Take heart from the fact that you will receive lots of visits from health care professionals over the first few days and don't be afraid to ask questions however silly you may think they are. I found I still had my pregnancy-brain on and so I wrote down anything I wanted to ask as I thought of it so I didn't forget.

- You will most likely be feeling tired, emotional and may have stitches, blood loss or other physical symptoms to recover from. Take time to do so and don't feel pressurised to return to your normal routine of cooking and cleaning too soon. A few dirty dishes and a messy front room pale into insignificance compared to the amazing gift you are experiencing of bonding with your baby.

- This is such a memorable time, why not add to your video diary if you have been keeping one. We got Samsara to leave a message for Cole and added ones of our own, as well as hours of footage of Cole doing a multitude of those brilliant baby things that entertain parents everywhere.

Things that I wish
I had known beforehand

- How to bath a baby and make sure that he was totally dry before putting a nappy on.
  It was a few days in before Dave and I realised that Cole had redness in the crease at the top of his legs which we could have prevented had we thought to gently pat the area dry with a soft cloth. Another area that can get sore is the neck where milk and dribble gather!

- Our doula told us about some fantastic ointment she used on all her children called 'Lucas Papaw Ointment'. It is from Australia and only contains fresh papaya and potassium sorbate, a preservative. Its many uses include helping relieve nappy rash, sore nipples and cracked skin. I eventually managed to buy some online but would have stocked up beforehand had I have known how useful it would be to us.

- Another great item that Samsara told us about was oversized muslins that you can use to swaddle your baby in. We struggled to contain Cole in the smaller cellular blankets we had bought - he would Houdini himself out after just a few minutes! I found a great company called 'Hamill Baby' that had absolutely gorgeous muslins in so many different designs and were a whopping 120cm square. We use ours to swaddle Cole, as a sun shade on his push chair and as sheets on his crib.

- We wished we had stocked up on clothes that were easy to put on a newborn. As novice parents we were incredibly cautious when dressing Cole and I subsequently favoured bodysuits that were of a cross-over style and didn't need to be pulled over his head. 'H&M' and 'Green Baby' always seem to have a large selection.

- This is going to sound strange but with the gift of hindsight I wished I had studied my boobs properly before I started breastfeeding. I had problems feeding Cole and ended up with very sore breasts. I was constantly asked by breastfeeding specialists, 'What did your nipples look like before you started feeding your baby?' and I honestly looked at my newly cracked, sore nipples and thought I don't remember but more importantly will they ever recover and return to normal?

  While I am on the subject of boobs I wish I had discovered sooner the marvellous bras made by 'Bravado' that are totally seamless. I ended up with mastitis quite early on when my bra and top left lines on my boobs that resulted in a redness and then full-on mastitis...ouch! Since I have been wearing the seamless bras I have avoided a repeat performance of it.

- I think that having a practice of changing a nappy on a real baby and also watching a mum breastfeeding would also have been invaluable to me.

- I also think that purchasing an electric breast pump, breastfeeding book and feeding cushion for Cole before he was born would have been better than leaving it until I was in a bit of a state with the whole breastfeeding lark!

- My final tip would be to buy a good baby book. I found an absolutely brilliant one called 'The Baby Book. Everything you need to know about your baby from birth to age two' by William and Martha Sears. I wish I had bought it before Cole's birth and had a good read up in advance. It has come to my rescue so many times and even my doctor commented on how good the advice in there was!

Meal planner

Monday

Breakfast: raspberry, banana and passion fruit smoothie, soya yoghurt, bran flakes, agave syrup, raisins and fresh blueberries

Snacks: rice cakes

Lunch: mixed leaf salad, beans, pasta and alfalfa with a tahini dressing

Snacks: coconut and dark chocolate bar

Dinner: veggie soya sausages, baked potato wedges and sweet potato in olive oil, and baked beans

Snack: fruit compote

Tuesday

Breakfast: seeds, puffed rice, and nut bar and a banana

Snacks: soya crisps

Lunch: wholegrain bread with houmous and salad and tofu cheesecake

Snacks: mixed nuts and raisins

Dinner: pasta with soya cream sauce, mushrooms, onion, garlic, courgettes, and fresh granary bread

Snacks: fruit soya yoghurt

Wednesday

Breakfast: pineapple, peach and passion fruit juice, wholemeal toast and cashew nut butter

Snack: mixed nuts and raisins

Lunch: rocket, peppers, cucumber, nutty potato salad, omega oil, linseed, hemp, and sesame seed sprinkles.

Snack: organic muesli bar

Dinner: brown basmati rice, sweet potatoes, butternut squash, mushrooms, onions and garlic in a coconut sauce

Snack: organic dark chocolate and almonds

Thursday

Breakfast: soya milk, cherry and banana smoothie, soya yoghurt, raisins, muesli, flaxseed, and agave syrup

Snack: wholemeal toast and mushroom pate

Lunch: avocado salad, lettuce, brazil nuts, cashew nuts, tomatoes, grated carrot with vegan mayonnaise, flaxseed oil and seeds

Snack: nut and puffed rice bar

Dinner: quinoa, red, yellow and green peppers, onions, nutritional yeast extract, cauliflower and broccoli with vegan soya cheese and milk sauce.

Snack: organic flapjack

Friday

Breakfast: coconut and banana smoothie, soya yoghurt, raisins, dried apricots, bran flakes, flaxseed powder, and agave syrup

Snack: homemade oat and dark chocolate cookies

Lunch: vegan spelt pizza with onion, peppers, olives, and vegan cheese with alfalfa, sprouting mung beans, flaxseed oil and seeds. Coleslaw with red cabbage, carrot, apple, walnuts and vegan mayonnaise

Dinner: brown rice, red lentil and walnut loaf with potatoes, sprouting broccoli, greens and gravy

Pudding: blackberry crumble with oats, desiccated coconut and vegan cream

Saturday

Breakfast: strawberry and banana smoothie, scrambled tofu and wholemeal toast with Marmite

Snack: nut bar

Lunch: sunflower seed bread with avocado, vegan 'bacon', tomato, cucumber, rocket, and alfalfa.

Snack: dried apricots, cranberries and brazil nuts

Dinner: brown rice, Chinese stir-fry with cashew nuts, tofu and soya sauce

Snack: fruit soya yoghurt

Sunday

Breakfast: pineapple, peach and passion fruit juice and a banana

Snack: wholegrain toast with cashew nut butter

Lunch: mixed leaf salad with chick peas, broccoli, cashew nuts, pine nuts, potatoes, olives, sweetcorn and alfalfa, dressed with vegan mayonnaise and omega oil (flaxseed and rapeseed)

Dinner: roast potatoes, soya sausages, 'cheatin turkey', carrots, cauliflower, and swede with gravy

Pudding: apple pie and vegan ice cream

My favourite suppliers and useful websites

For helpful information & advice

NHS Direct	www.nhsdirect.nhs.uk
Baby Centre	www.babycentre.co.uk
NCT	www.nctpregnancyandbabycare.com
Doula UK	www.doula.org.uk
Samsara Tanner - our doula	www.samsaradoula.co.uk
HypnoBirthing UK	www.hypnobirthing.co.uk
Karen Knight - HypnoBirthing Brighton	www.hypnobabes.co.uk
Homebirth Organisation	www.homebirth.org.uk
Homebirth group Brighton	www.brightonandhove-nct.org.uk/homebirth.htm
Vegan Society	www.vegansociety.com
Vegetarian Society	www.vegsoc.org
Boots baby club	www.boots.com/en/Mother-Baby/Parenting-Club/
Bounty Parenting Club	www.bounty.com

For lotions and potions to see you through your pregnancy

Neal's Yard Remedies	www.nealsyardremedies.com
Mama Mio	www.mamamio.com
Sanctuary mum-to-be range	www.thesanctuary.co.uk/mum-to-be.htm

Maternity and breastfeeding clothes

JoJo Maman Bébé	www.jojomamanbebe.co.uk
Blooming Marvellous	www.bloomingmarvellous.co.uk
Yummy Mummy Maternity	www.yummymummymaternity.co.uk
Mothercare	www.mothercare.com
MumsTheWord	www.mumstheword.com

Birth Pools

The Good Birth Company	www.thegoodbirth.co.uk

Clothes, essentials & goodies for you and your baby

Mothercare	www.mothercare.com
Boots	www.boots.com
JoJo Maman Bébé	www.jojomamanbebe.co.uk
MumsTheWord	www.mumstheword.com
Green Baby	www.greenbaby.co.uk
Yummies	www.yummies.biz
Lili may	www.lilimay.com
Cath Kidston	www.cathkidston.co.uk

Marks & Spencer	www.marksandspencer.com
Hamill Baby - large muslins & more	www.hamillbaby.com
Little Green Earthlets - nappies & more	www.earthlets.co.uk
Spirit of Nature Eco-disposable nappies	www.spiritofnature.co.uk
Lucas Papaw Ointment	www.pawpawstore.co.uk
Symphony in Motion, cot mobile	www.tinylove.com
Weleda - Baby massage oil	www.weleda.co.uk
Earth Friendly Baby - wipes	www.earthfriendlybaby.com
Baby sun-lotion, shampoo & body wash	www.greenpeople.co.uk

AVAILABLE NOW...

The True Diary of a Bride-to-be

Something blue for the Bride-to-be

When Charlie was little, a gypsy fortune teller at a village fair told her when she grew up she would be married twice...

Now fast forward to some thirty years later in Paris, where her boyfriend unexpectedly pops the big question.

In Charlie's diary she shares her experiences and insights as she plans for not just one wedding, but two - to the same man!

From the bright lights of Vegas to a whirlwind honeymoon around America, and back home in time for wedding number two at the beautiful Royal Pavilion in Brighton.

Her diary is a true account of exactly how she planned for each wedding without losing the plot. At the end of each week she focuses on tips and things to do to help ensure that you too will have the wedding of your dreams.

The True Diary of a Bride-to-be includes:

- Ideas on where, when and how to host the most amazing wedding.

- Little reminders to help you keep on top of managing your finances.

- Weekly guides on practicalities such as how to find the perfect people to support you on your big day.

- Finding the perfect dress and accessories.

- The fun bits, including sampling food and wine.

- Tips on how to keep your own special journal, memory box or scrapbook.

Coming soon....

The True Diary of Baby's first year

In Charlie's Diary she recounts those magical first days when she finally gains access to the best club in the world 'Parenthood'...

Her diary is a humorous and honest account of her attempts to be that ever elusive 'Yummy Mummy' she keeps reading about. But with boobs that are so sore getting fully dressed isn't really an option and no free time to visit a hairdressers she finds that 'Scummy Mummy' may be a more accurate description of herself!...

Join Charlie in her adventures in 'Baby Land' as she learns that with perseverance, love and support from her husband and those around her that she has got what it takes to be the scrumiest yummiest mummy in town!

The True Diary of Baby's First Year includes:

- Tips for regaining your figure, taking care of yourself and your baby.

- A weekly guide to your baby's development.

- Fun things to do with your baby to help with the bonding process.

- Recommended products you will utilise again and again.

- Ideas for keeping your own baby journal, photo book and time tin.

Lightning Source UK Ltd.
Milton Keynes UK
27 January 2011

166474UK00001B/20/P